Doctor, Matilda's in Labor!

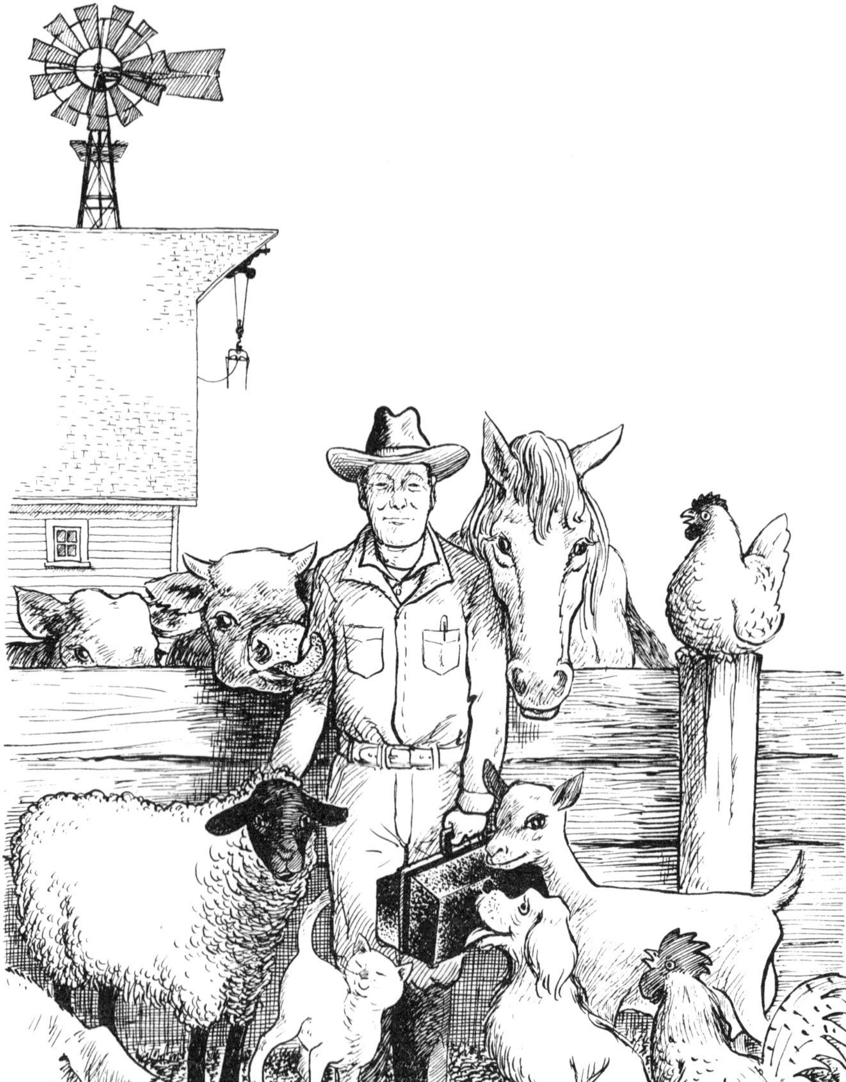
BOB ARTLEY '85

Doctor, Matilda's in Labor!

by JAMES A. PORTER, JR., D.V.M., M.P.H., Ph.D.

Iowa State University Press, Ames

Dedicated to the Memory of My Father *Dr. Armer Porter,*
Who Taught Me How to Vet

First Edition, 1986

Library of Congress Cataloging-in-Publication Data

Porter, James A. (James Armer), 1922-
Doctor, Matilda's in labor!

1. Porter, James A. (James Armer), 1922- . 2. Veterinarians—Kansas—Fredonia—Biography. 3. Fredonia (Kan.)—Biography. I. Title.
SF613.P6A34 1986 636.089'092'4 [B] 85-23875
ISBN 0-8138-0463-9

Contents

Preface

I was born October 8, 1922 at Fredonia, Kansas. My father, Dr. Armer Porter, was a student at Kansas State College in Manhattan, Kansas, at the time of my birth. He had returned to college after serving in France during World War I. A bullet shattered his kneecap during the Battle of the Argonne and left him permanently crippled. The government sent him to college to rehabilitate him on a "GI Bill." He had been a farmer previously and took veterinary medicine as an alternative vocation. After his graduation in 1925, he returned to his home town of Fredonia to practice.

Although his proper name was James Armer Porter, he went by the name of Armer Porter. My given name was James Armer Porter, Jr., but I went by the name Armer Porter, Jr., while going through school in Fredonia. My relatives and Armer's peers called me Junior. My classmates called me "Doc" because of my father's vocation.

After graduation from Fredonia High School in 1940, I matriculated at Kansas State College in veterinary medicine to follow in my father's footsteps. For various reasons I started going by the name of James Porter or Jimmy at college. After graduation I shortened the Jimmy to Jim. This explains the different names I use in referring to myself in the text.

In December 1941 the United States entered World War II and my life, as well as the life of my contemporaries, was permanently changed. I was "frozen" in college and placed on an accelerated schedule. The veterinary corps was filled by the time I graduated in May 1944, so I worked in the U.S. Meat Inspection Service and the U.S. Maritime Service. In August 1945 I returned to Fredonia to practice with my father.

Fredonia, a rural town of some three thousand people, is on the dividing line between the area of small family farms and the big cattle ranches that stretch up through the Flint Hills pasture area of east central Kansas. The practice was primarily cattle and hogs; however, the Porters were the only veterinarians in the county, so we provided service to any animal or bird presented.

I worked with my father out of a house that served as an office next to my father's residence until 1947, when I went to Mexico to work with the U.S. Department of Agriculture on the program to eradicate foot-and-mouth disease from that country. When I returned to Fredonia in 1949, I opened up a veterinary office with corral, restraint facilities, and the like, for a truck-in veterinary practice. Later, I moved to a similar office adjoining the local livestock sales barn, facing the fair grounds. My uncle, Ed Gillies, served in my office at my first location; Ceres Sell served at the second location. Clarence Fateley joined me as an assistant in handling animals for the last ten years I was in Fredonia. They have all died but I am eternally grateful for their loyal service. In addition, Dr. Jim Smart assisted me during my last year in practice.

I have changed names of most other persons except relatives and some faculty members. I have also changed certain facts so that outsiders will not be able to identify the parties involved. Many of the people have died. Others, though, still live in the area and will recognize incidents and persons. I have not meant to say anything derogatory about any person and wish to apologize if any person resents anything I have written about them. I still love them all.

I was raised in Fredonia during the Great Depression. Our area suffered severe droughts several times during the thirties. Fredonia was east of the Dust Bowl, but I remember many a day when the dust blew through with visibility restricted to one hundred yards or less. Most of the farm houses had been built by homesteaders after the Civil War. The rural homes were without electricity and inside plumbing, and radios were operated by batteries. Conditions were primitive by today's standards, but we knew no different.

After World War II, the Rural Electrification Administration sponsored a program to provide electricity to the rural areas. Bathrooms were built onto or into houses. Farms became larger. Many small farmers worked part or full time off the farm. New houses were constructed. The area was in a state of transition when I practiced.

My father and I worked with primitive laboratory facilities. Although I had a portable chute, a large animal operating table, corrals, and the like, we did not have an X-ray machine or any of the other diagnostic equipment considered essential today except a microscope. We relied primarily on our senses to make diagnoses.

The times and events described are a vanishing part of Americana and are written with the hope of preserving a bit of this heritage.

Doctor, Matilda's in Labor!

Father Goes to College

My father was a veterinarian in the small rural town of Fredonia, Kansas, while I was growing up. Although my nickname was "Doc" because of my father, I never seriously considered becoming a veterinarian until my senior year in high school. My father's life was physically demanding, required long hours, and didn't offer sufficient financial returns to attract me. Since I participated in public speaking activities while in high school, my mother thought I would decide on law or, better yet, enter the ministry. My thoughts didn't coincide with my mother's. I certainly couldn't feature myself in the pulpit chastising the parishioners for their sins. I was undecided about what to do until my senior year, when I became attracted by the positions the government was offering to veterinarians. After experiencing the hardships of the depression of the 1930s and seeing my father accept eggs, meat, and other farm produce in lieu of cash, the security of a government job seemed attractive. Accordingly, I enrolled at Kansas State College (now Kansas State University), as my father had twenty years before to get a veterinary education.

I had been exposed to college at an early age. Although born in Fredonia, I spent the first three years of my life at Manhattan, Kansas, the location of Kansas State College, while my father completed his college education. He had been wounded during World War I. A machine-gun bullet shattered his left kneecap, leaving him with a stiff knee and a limp for the rest of his life. To rehabilitate him for work he was physically capable of doing, the government provided him with a "GI Bill" to return to school. He had been a farmer. He chose to study to become a veterinarian. In those days all veterinarians worked with horses. Why the government, or my father for that matter, thought that the life of a "horse doctor" would be physically easier than that of a farmer, I don't know. Nevertheless, after his return from France, he and my mother moved to Manhattan so he could start his education.

His prior education had been limited to attending a one-room brick school that provided no education past the eighth grade—all grades being taught by one teacher. Nowadays there would be some law or labor regulation to prevent this, but my father's generation considered that a teacher with one or two years of normal school education was capable. In addition to salary, the teachers received board and room. In my father's school district, Rock Creek, the teacher was boarded at his parents' house. That was the way my father met my mother. It was also the way most of father's brothers met their wives. Thus my mother and some of my aunts on my father's side had one thing in common. They had taught at Rock Creek School and had boarded at the Porter's house.

Therefore, with only an eighth grade education, my father faced the necessity of getting a high school education before he could enter veterinary school. So he enrolled at Manhattan High School. My mother recounted stories of my father coming home from school with test papers and compositions marked A and being just as tickled as his teenage classmates were. I suspect that she may have helped write many of the compositions and thus shared in his elation at receiving an A. He finished four years of high school in two years. He then applied for and was accepted into veterinary school. Four years later he graduated near the top of his class with honors. That there were only seven persons in the class did not detract from the honor. Unfortunately, this was the standard that I was to be judged against. This might not have been so bad except that many of his professors of twenty years before were there to do the judging—but there were also compensations.

One of the professors was "Daddy Burt." Dr. Burt was nearing retirement when I knew him. He had taught forty years and still remembered each of his former students. He had a warm spot in his heart for Armer, my father. They were about the same age so had been somewhat closer than professor and student. To him, I was Armer's boy and he always asked about Armer when I returned from a holiday trip home. One advantage this may have had was to enable me to win a five dollar bet in the days when the dollar was still worth something. The second semester in veterinary school required that half the credit load, eight hours, be in anatomy. This was the last semester that I had the opportunity to take a minimum of sixteen hours—but I'm digressing from the story. A classmate bet me that I couldn't earn an A in the eight hours of anatomy. Although I memorized Sisson's *Anatomy,* it was probably nip and tuck as to whether I earned an A or B. Dr. Burt gave me an A. I have always felt that Dr. Burt's friendship for my father may have influenced a borderline decision, but that didn't deter me from collecting the five dollars. This was one example of how the respect and friendship the professors had for my father may have aided me.

Anatomy, as taught in those days, was based on the horse. During the previous decade the tractor had replaced the horse as a means of power. During this transition period there was talk of the veterinary profession becoming unneeded. However, because of the growing value of food animals and the growing importance of pet animals in people's lives, the decade of the thirties closed with a strong resurgence of interest in veterinary medicine that continues to increase to this day. Because textbooks are often several years behind current developments, we still studied Sisson's *Anatomy,* which was primarily based on the horse. To update the book, small supplemental sections on the cow, pig, dog, and chicken had been added. Dissections in the laboratory were based on the horse. There was an economic reason for this. Horses were relatively cheap; they had been used for years, so why change? We spent many hours weekly, in a laboratory reeking with formalin, dissecting equine cadavers suspended from the overhead rails. For every class the cadavers were rolled out of the cooler to the students' stations. Every day, at the conclusion of class, the cadavers were rolled back into the cooler, still reeking with the preservative, to await the next class period.

Another professor was Dr. E. J. Frick, director of clinics. He didn't realize I was Armer's son until my senior year in veterinary school. Porter is a common name and there were three other Porters, none related to me, in veterinary school at the same time I was there. He finally recognized me as Armer's son when, as a class assignment, I turned in plans for a veterinary hospital for Dr. Armer Porter.

"Porter, are you Armer Porter's son?"

"Yes. Why?"

"Gee, I didn't realize I was getting old until I realized that I have former students sending their sons back to study. How is Armer?"

My father knew Dr. Frick when he first arrived in Manhattan to teach. He had graduated from Cornell University and was fresh out of the army veterinary corps. To my father, he was still a Broadway cowboy who didn't quite fit into the rural Kansas scene. Dr. Frick changed during the twenty intervening years before I arrived at veterinary school. He lost his New York attitudes and became an integral part of the college staff dedicated to educating veterinarians who have left their stamp on the profession. Students had respect tempered with fear for Dr. Frick. He ruled the clinics with a tight fist. Everyone had daily assignments. If a student finished his assignments, it behooved him to find something to keep him busy. If not, Dr. Frick would catch him and put him to work preparing drugs for the pharmacy, or exercising animals, or mowing grass in the paddocks. He would catch the unwary by asking for volunteers who could type. The eager beavers who raised their hands were put to work shoveling manure from the stable. One of my classmates claimed that he made it a point to walk fast with a preoccupied look on his face whenever he saw Dr. Frick approaching so that he would have the appearance of being busy. I had difficulty in assuming the right facial expression.

When things slackened during the afternoon, Dr. Frick would assemble those not busy in the amphitheater and deliver lectures. These could cover anything from clinical practice to identifying breeds of dogs, to practical business, to politics, or to anything that was on Dr. Frick's mind that day. We were a captive audience and Dr. Frick loved it. Some years after I graduated, a senior class presented him with an award. It was a gilded trophy of a man grasping a bull by the rear leg and swinging it around over his head. On the pedestal of the trophy was a metal plate with the words "The Champion Bull Thrower" engraved upon it. Although initially Dr. Frick was somewhat taken aback by the receipt of this award, he rapidly regained his composure. Later he delighted in taking former students returning to the campus up to his office to exhibit the trophy.

Professor John Wilson left an indelible impression on the students. Fortunately for my father, he arrived after his time. Dr. Wilson was finishing a Ph.D. in parasitology but was teaching histology. His students both feared and hated him. To me, his special talent seemed to be to make the subject matter of a lecture completely unintelligible to the ordinary mortal and to act as a "guillotine" in flunking out the undesirable students—or, at least, the students he felt to be undesirable. I never understood what he was saying in his lectures so I didn't know whether he was a genius or just a poor lecturer. He gave exams that had questions with as many as twenty-five multiple choice answers—any, all, or none of which might be correct. His grading system on these exams was something that might have come out of Dante's *Inferno.* A person could easily, and often did, get a minus score. He claimed his type of examinations discouraged guessing. One of my classmates claimed he did as well by going out on a beer bust the night before so that his brain wouldn't be cluttered with scientific trivia as he randomly marked answers on the exam. A fifty or better was an A. I passed one of his courses with a D, the only D I ever received in college, and I was happy to receive it.

After he finished his Ph.D., Dr. Wilson moved to another university to teach parasitology. In later years I too received a Ph.D. in parasitology. Judicious inquiries of colleagues indicated he was well thought of by his students at this university. His problem at Kansas State may have been due to teaching in a field that was not his main interest, or it may have been immaturity in developing teaching skills, or it may have been our attitude towards his course. Whatever the reason, many of my classmates have bitter memories of their exposure to him.

Many years later, when I was in graduate school, I had to get a background in histology. I learned this on the side from a professor and friend at the University of Illinois. Until that time I had the feeling that histology was an occult science taught by demons armed with pitchforks ready to remove unsuspecting and helpless students from veterinary school.

Dr. L. D. Bushnell was an "old timer," who taught bacteriology. My classmates and I were amazed at his fund of knowledge in this field. In reply to an inquiry from a classmate, he explained that the reason he knew so much was that there were only three bacteria known when he started studying in this field. When I was in school there were hundreds and now there are thousands.

During one of his exams my textbook fell to the floor. A deadly silence fell over the class as everybody, including Dr. Bushnell, watched me bend over and pick up the open book. The next day I received in my mail box a notice from Dr. Bushnell's office informing me that I had flunked the exam because of opening a text in class.

"Jim, what have you got there?" Ray asked solicitously.

"Say, that's a failure notice, isn't it?" John chimed in.

"What's it in? Oh, Bushnell's course. I told you not to try to look at a book during his quizzes. He's flunked students before on that."

"But I didn't try to look at the book. It was an accident, it dropped."

"Well, if you say so, but Dr. Bushnell will never believe you."

"You can repeat the course next year if the draft doesn't pick you up, Jim." (The year was 1941 and a selective service draft for military service was operating.)

"Shucks, Jim, you may like the army. It might be better than coming back here."

"But I don't want to go to the army."

"We don't always have a choice. You can't get a deferment working for your father, can you? Maybe he could claim he needs you in his practice just to assist."

"My draft board wouldn't buy that."

"Well, you won't have to leave for a few days. We'll have a farewell party for you before you go."

I didn't want a farewell party. I wanted to stay in school. How should I approach Dr. Bushnell? Maybe, if I waited a day or two, his anger would subside. After spending an uneasy day and a sleepless night, I found myelf still undecided.

Ray approached me the next morning. "Jim, did you sleep well?"

"Not very. Why?"

"Well, one of your classmates, who prefers to remain anonymous, told me to tell you that he stole that flunk slip blank from Dr. Bushnell's office. You really didn't receive a flunk slip."

"What?"

"You didn't flunk—unless you flunked the exam. But we still want to have a party for you. We'll call it a "Welcome Back Party."

"Thanks."

I was so relieved I didn't even push to learn my colleague's name. Besides, I would probably be on the other end the next time.

Physiology lab was another place for pranks. One of the tests required was to determine the presence or absence of sugar in the urine. The presence of a high level indicated diabetes. We used our own urine for the test. One of my classmates did indeed have an extremely positive urine.

"Gee, Jack, how do you feel?"

"Well, I guess I haven't been feeling well for the last few months. I've been too upset to study at nights. Is that a sign of diabetes?"

"It must be. The rest of us have no trouble studying. Maybe if you'll start taking insulin, you can settle down and study. Did you ever have to inject yourself?"

"No. Does it hurt?"

"They say the hardest part is being brave enough to stick a needle into yourself. I don't know if I could do it."

"Maybe I can get Jim to do it at first."

"Jack, I think you'd better do it yourself. We can get some tuberculin needles over at the clinic and you can practice on yourself. You inject yourself in the legs rather than the arms anyway. That way people won't think you are a junkie."

"Before you people get to jabbing too many needles into yourselves, you had better run another test." It was Dr. Roger Link speaking. "I think I saw someone leaving the room with a sack of sugar in his hand."

"That S.O.B. I'll get him tonight."

Few changes had occurred in the twenty years between the student days of my father and myself. An old three-story limestone building that served as a classroom and office building and the adjoining limestone building that served as a hospital were the same. The number of faculty may have increased from ten to twenty, but considering that the classes had increased in size as much as tenfold, this was an insignificant increase. Laboratory equipment was still largely restricted to microscopes and X-ray machines. Treatments taught were largely the same. Few new drugs had entered the field. Sulfa was now being used and reports on a new medicine, penicillin, were being heard. Intravenous barbiturate anesthetics replaced inhalation anesthetics such as ether. One of the few miracle drugs that had entered everyday use was an injectable calcium drug that was now used to treat "milk fever" in cows, replacing the former method that consisted of pumping air into the quarters of the udder. Because of the lack of miracle drugs for most conditions, my father emphasized to me the importance of learning the toxic dose of drugs—his reasoning being that if you didn't kill the animal with the medicine, nature would see to the healing of most conditions.

I recently returned to Kansas State for the thirty-fifth class reunion and for the dedication of a new veterinary complex. At the dedication I toured a new three-building campus that had fifty times as many square feet of space as the buildings that my father and I attended. The faculty had grown to over seventy-five persons. Laboratories and clinic were equipped with all types of monitoring and testing equipment that were never dreamed of in either my father's or my student days. Veterinary medicine had become a science as well as an art.

Pearl Harbor Day (December 7, 1941) occurred during my freshman year of veterinary school. This greatly influenced my life as it did the lives of millions of other people. In my case, it resulted in a phobia for classrooms, brought on by overexposure. At the completion of the freshman year in veterinary school, my classmates and I were "frozen" in school and placed on an accelerated course. We finished the last three years of school in two years. We attended classes from 7:00 A.M. until 5:00 P.M., six days a week, twelve months a year, except for one six-week free period the first summer. After 5:00 P.M., we were supposed to find time to study for a course load running from 30 to 50 percent above normal. Most of us managed to graduate, possibly because our professors sympathized with our plight. By the last year in school, I had developed a phobia for classroooms. I just wanted to graduate. I didn't want to ever enter a classroom again.

"Marian, I Couldn't Get a Marriage License"

After completing my first year of college and working during the summer before I entered the second year of veterinary college, I had to find another rooming house after school had begun. So I moved in with three of my classmates, Ray Parker, Harry Owens, and Dave Smith. They were living in a three-story house, with the family living on the first floor. The upper two floors had been rented out to students. Somehow, the upper floor had been taken over by ladies catering to the lusts of the soldiers at the nearby military bases. Most of the former male student occupants moved out, leaving the four of us with the occupancy of the entire second floor. Actually, it was an ideal arrangement for us except on weekend nights. At that time the soldiers would come up the front stairs and walk down the second floor hallway, peering into our rooms as they went. They had questioning looks on their faces when they saw us. Somehow, they were expecting something different. We seldom said a word; we just pointed down the hallway towards the rear stairs going up to the third floor. Sometimes on a Saturday or Sunday morning our second floor bathroom might look a little the worse for overuse by the third floor visitors, but overall it was a comfortable arrangement that was to continue until the college housing authority found out what was going on and made us evacuate.

While living there, Harry and I became enamored of the two girls we later married. They were college students like ourselves, so most of our socializing during the week was confined to library dates. On weekends we would take in a dance or a movie. Actually, there was little other choice. One of the events of the season was the "Gold Digger's Ball." The girls had the opportunity to select dates and take them to the ball. Jan and Marian, our respective girlfriends, asked us to the ball.

"Now you boys must meet us down at the corner. We're not coming to the door. Some soldier might mistake us for one of the creatures upstairs."

"What creatures upstairs?"

"You know what we're talking about. You meet us at the corner."

"Oh, we'll be ready. We won't leave you stranded on the porch. Ring the bell. We'll come right down."

The girls were hesitant about the arrangement but agreed. Harry and I came up with the idea that we ought to embellish our front porch by exchanging a red light bulb for the frosted white bulb in the ceiling on the evening of our dates. At the arranged hour, Jan and Marian came down the street to pick us up. As they neared the house, they saw the red light.

"Jan, do you see what I see?"

"That is their porch, isn't it?"

"I knew we shouldn't agree to pick them up. I'm not going up there with that red light shining on me."

"Me neither."

Twenty minutes later Ray came up to our room to inform us that Jan and Marian were waiting down at the corner, and if we wanted them to take us to the "Gold Digger's Ball," we had better come down to the corner to meet them. Harry and I decided that we had played the red light stunt for all it was worth so put on our coats and went to meet our dates.

The following spring Marian and I decided to get married. I wasn't getting enough studying done on library dates and the course schedule seemed to be getting heavier. Getting married seemed to be the answer if I was to get my mind back on my studies and graduate. Marian, at that time, was a resident dietitian student at Van Zile Hall (a girls' residence hall). The professor in charge frowned on having married dietitian residents—possibly the result of an unhappy affair that she had personally experienced. Anyway, Marian believed that it would be better if the marriage was not publicized until after she received her diploma that spring. Marian's parents were working in Canada and knew nothing of what was occurring. Easter came later that year. We planned to take advantage of the extra day off from school to get married and to spend our honeymoon in Kansas City. Marian couldn't get away from the dormitory until Saturday morning that weekend, so I went to Kansas City on Friday to arrange for the marriage license. I found out after arrival in Kansas City that licenses could only be issued if representatives of both parties were present. They wouldn't issue the license to me by myself. I had to get a representative for Marian. I telephoned a cousin who lived in Kansas City for assistance.

"Eiliene, this is Armer, Jr." My relatives knew me as Armer, Jr.

"Well, hello. Where are you calling from?"

"I'm in town."

"Can you come out? Cecil will be home by five."

"Well, I'm uptown and need some help."

"What kind of help?"

"I need help getting a marriage license."

"A what?"

"A marriage license."

"For who?"

"For me. My fiancée can't get to town until tomorrow and I have to have her or a stand-in to get a license today before the office closes for the weekend."

"You mean you're getting married?"

"Yes, if I can get a license."

"Do your parents know about this?"

"Not yet."

"What do you think Aunt Sybil and Uncle Armer will say?"

"Oh, they won't care. I just haven't gotten around to telling them yet."

"I don't know about this."

"Eiliene, I need your help up here to stand in as a proxy for my fiancée to get this license today."

"I don't know your fiancée."

"Her name is Marian Oldham. I'll introduce you when she gets to town tomorrow."

"I don't know, besides I haven't any way to get to town this afternoon."

"There's a bus, isn't there?"

"Yes, but I can't leave my two children."

"Can't you get a baby sitter?"

"Not at this hour."

"Well, bring them along."

"I can't drag them uptown. Besides it would look a little peculiar for me to be getting a marriage license with two children tagging along."

"You won't be getting the license. You'll be a proxy. I need your help if I get married this weekend."

"Maybe you ought to think about this over the weekend. Doesn't Marian have any relatives or friends here that can help?"

"Yes, but she doesn't want them to know."

"Why? If she doesn't want them to know, I don't think I had better get involved."

"O.K." I was getting no place. Dejectedly I hung up. Things were in a mess.

I met Marian and her bridesmaid, Betty Butler, when they arrived on the train at Union Station Saturday morning.

"See, I did show up. When are we getting married?"

"I didn't get a license."

"You didn't get a license? You changed your mind?"

"No, that isn't it at all." I explained the problem. "What are we going to do'"

"I came here to get married. I expect to get married."

"We can't get a license until Monday. School starts on Tuesday."

"I guess I can stay over until Tuesday to go back. I came to get married. I'm not going back until I get married. I'm still worried about my supervisor at Van Zile finding out about me getting married. Let's take a train to an adjoining county on Monday to get the license and get married. That way it won't appear in the *Kansas City Star* and she'll never know about it."

"O.K. I guess I can miss class Tuesday morning. The wedding is on."

Betty arranged to rejoin us on Monday. Marian made arrangements to stay at an aunt's home on Saturday and Sunday nights—she never enlightened them on her wedding plans. No need to have the word passed back to her parents and have the monthly subsistence checks cut off with only three months to go until graduation. I spent the next two nights alone in a room at the Hotel Continental.

On Monday morning Marian, Betty, and I met at the Union Station and I purchased round-trip tickets to the town of Warrensburg, located in an adjoining county. The schedules were such that we could get there and back the same day with enough time to take care of the legalities and the ceremony.

"Do you still want to go through with it?" Marian asked. "You won't have an excuse today like you came up with Saturday."

"I bought the train tickets, didn't I? Besides, I'm getting lonesome in the hotel room by myself."

"Well, we certainly don't want you to get lonesome," Betty interjected. "Let's get the knot tied. They're calling our train now."

We fell in with hundreds of other persons walking down the train platform looking for a passenger car with empty seats. Those were the days of gasoline and tire rationing. Trains were the primary means of transportation and every train was filled to capacity. Every car was filled by the persons ahead of us before we arrived. Finally, in desperation, we pushed into a car already filled. We had come this far; we had to get to Warrensburg today. Although there were no empty seats, Marian and Betty managed to sit down by improvising the suitcase Marian was carrying as a seat at the end of the car. Marian had said goodbye to her aunt that morning, telling her she was returning to Manhattan. She would carry the suitcase to Warrensburg and then back to our hotel later that day. I braced myself next to Marian and stood swaying with the movement of the car as we made the trip to Warrensburg.

In Warrensburg we took a taxi to the county courthouse. This time there were no problems in securing the license. The only irregularity was that I lied about my age. I lacked a few months of being twenty-one but stated I was twenty-one to secure the license. The clerk took my word for it. Though procuring a marriage license using false information might be grounds for annulment, neither Marian nor her parents ever made the effort. Now, after forty years, I presume that the "grandfather clause" or some other regulation would be in effect and that nobody could declare the marriage illegal. With this presumption I can now rest easy that my children will not be declared illegitimate by some court of law and that I can go to my grave with a clear conscience. At the time I was willing to gamble on falsifying the record. The hotel room was too expensive for single occupancy, and I was lonesome in the room by myself.

After receiving the license I telephoned the local pastor of our faith. He was home and would be happy to marry us. We walked the two blocks to the manse of Reverend Jack Smith, minister of the local Disciples of Christ congregation. Marian, assisted by Betty, stepped into a bedroom to change into her wedding suit while I exchanged pleasantries with Reverend Smith. In a few minutes Marian and Betty rejoined us and Marian and I exchanged vows in a simple ceremony. It wasn't elaborate. It didn't match the pomp and ceremony of many other weddings I have attended, including that of my eldest daughter; however, it did take—at least for forty years.

When we returned to Kansas City, we parted from Betty and I finally took my bride to the hotel. I changed the register from my name to that of Mr. and Mrs. James Porter to the knowing smiles of the clerk. That night, our doorknob was rattled and the pipes of the radiator were pounded intermittently all night long, presumably by the bell boys wishing us well.

Several of my classmates got married during the next few months; presumably all were twenty-one years of age. I was the only one living in sin. Two couples, Jan and Harry, now married, and Marian and I, accompanied one of the newlywed couples on their honeymoon trip to Kansas City. They were fortunate to have a car, so the reason for our presence was to act as chauffeurs and chaperones as far as Kansas City. After that they would be on their own. The car they were driving had the usual "Just Married" sign painted on it. When we pulled up in front of the Hotel Continental a crowd quickly gathered to see the blushing bride. Marian and I jumped out and embraced before the applauding crowd. Sue and Tom, the newlyweds, made their escape into the hotel lobby while the rest of us retrieved our suitcases, saw to the parking of the car, and dispersed for the weekend.

That summer, after Marian finished her residency at Van Zile Hall, we moved into a basement apartment and started living as man and wife. By that time we had informed both sets of parents and were not disowned. We were both working, Marian full time, so finances were no major problem. A group of us married or soon-to-be-married couples picnicked and played bridge together. School was forgotten as much as possible.

One evening we were picnicking at Sunset Park with some friends. Marian and I were walking along a trail near the stream and I was ahead of her. A branch hung down over the trail and I pulled it out of the way. I didn't realize how close Marian was and released the branch at the wrong moment. It sprang back and caught her over the eye causing a very black and blue facial swelling.

"Jim, you've been fighting with Marian already?" Cal asked.

"I wasn't fighting. It was a branch of a tree at Sunset."

"Now, Jim, all married people have problems. You don't need to lie to me. I'm your friend."

"Cal, I was walking ahead of Marian . . ."

"Jim, the fight wasn't serious, was it? You won't be getting a divorce, will you?"

"Cal, I'm trying to tell you what happened."

"I would rather you hadn't done that now. I was getting ready to propose to Marie. She may think twice after seeing that eye of Marian's."

"Cal, don't you think you have some place where you have to go?"

That fall Marian decided to take some advanced dietetic training with the federal government in Washington, D.C., while I was finishing my schooling. I moved over to the Bakers' and shared a room with Cal. One night I received a telephone call from Marian's parents.

"Jim, we're in Kansas City for a couple of days on our way to Florida. We'd like to see you."

"Fine. I'll give you my address. Come on over."

"I'm afraid we don't have time or transportation. We would sure like you to come down and see us. We are here at the Aladin Hotel."

"I don't know if I can get off. I have a heavy class schedule."

"I'm sure you can get off. We'll be looking for you tomorrow night."

"Well, if I can get off."

Ethel Baker had overheard the conversation. "That was Marian's parents wasn't it?"

"Yes. They want me to come to Kansas City to meet them."

"You're going, aren't you?"

"I don't think so. I don't have time."

"Jim, you've got time. They are Marian's parents."

"I don't see why they can't come here."

"Jim, it is appropriate for the prospective groom to ask the father for his daughter's hand. Since you did away with some of the formalities, it would be proper for you to go to Kansas City now and pay your respects."

The next day I was on the highway hitchhiking into Kansas City to meet the parents. It would probably have been easier to have asked Frank for Marian's hand beforehand rather than to meet the two of them now without Marian to run interference. What if they found out I wasn't twenty-one years old? What if they wanted to annul the marriage?

That evening I met them at their hotel room.

"Jim, I'm DeArcy and this is Frank."

"How do you do."

"We're doing fine. How is Marian? How are you? When do you finish? What are you and Marian going to do then?" The questions came one after the other.

I found the meeting wasn't as dreadful as I feared. They never asked my age. They never seemed critical of our running off and getting married. They never hinted at annulment. It wasn't nearly as bad as I thought it would be. If I had known this, I would have gotten married years ago—that is, if I had been twenty-one years of age.

Frank had been in my hometown, Fredonia, on many occasions. He used to be a traveling salesman and traveled from one town to the other in the central part of the United States. He sold shoes when he traveled through Fredonia. In later years, Frank had taken a correspondence course in law. Florida was one of the few states still permitting correspondence school graduates to take the bar examination. He had passed the exam in Florida a few years previously and was now returning from work in Canada on the Alcan Highway office staff to start a practice in Miami. They hoped Marian and I would come to see them, and they would be delighted if we moved to Miami after the war was over. After a delightful evening, I retired. In-laws weren't as bad as they were made out to be. Ethel was right. It was right for me to go to Kansas City to meet Marian's parents.

During a break between classes in the fall, I hitchhiked to Washington to see Marian. She wasn't happy with her job. It involved clean-up activities. It did not involve preparing foods. A month after I returned to Manhattan, Marian quit and returned to Manhattan to join me. We moved into an apartment above Slim's to be near the action and the restaurant where I worked.

One of the problems of preparing for a dance in Kansas was to make the liquor, hard to come by in a "dry" state, go as far as possible. Since we had an apartment near the social activities center, our friends flocked in to help prepare the "purple passion" for the evening's refreshment. A bottle of vodka with several cans of fruit juice used as an extender would make the evening for a large party. When we were fortunate, we dispensed with the vodka and used alcohol from the college pharmacy.

"Bill, did you get the alcohol?"

"I never fail. Here it is."

"Now this is ethyl, isn't it?"

"Jim, you know I wouldn't pan off any methyl on you."

"Bill, how do you manage to get this?"

"Well, I won't tell anyone else but since you're married, I'll tell you. The girl who manages the pharmacy storeroom has a crush on me."

"What about Margaret?"

"You've heard about sailors who have a girl in every port, haven't you?"

"Sure."

"Well, I'm like that except I have a girl in every department."

"This is a small campus. What are you going to do if they find out about each other?"

"Jim, don't mention it. The evening is beautiful. Margaret is really passionate tonight. Don't drag in ugly thoughts."

"Well, if push comes to shove, keep in good with the girl in the pharmacy storeroom or turn her over to one of our colleagues. We do need the ethyl. I don't have enough vodka to carry us through to graduation."

"Jim, don't sweat it. There's ten girls for every single man on campus now. We can always get alcohol."

Kansas State's enrollment was reduced from a prewar number of seven to eight thousand to a 1944 figure of around sixteen hundred, most of the number being girls, 4F male students, or uniformed students. College social activities as known today did not exist under those circumstances. There were Saturday night dances and married couples got together to play bridge or picnic; however, there was little overall to detract from our main purpose of finishing our education as fast as possible.

I had three things to prepare for. I had to pass my finals in my classwork so I could get my diploma. I had to prepare to take my accreditation examination for the federal government. I had to prepare to take the state boards in veterinary medicine in Kansas and any other state in which I had an interest. Being married kept me home far more than previously and I managed to get through even though the classrooms themselves became a phobia to me, as mentioned previously—a phobia that I didn't overcome for sixteen years.

Commencement exercises were one of the memorable events of my life. I had finished my training for adulthood—at least I thought I had. My grandmother Short and my parents sat with Marian in the auditorium as I marched across the stage and, with a wide grin on my face, eagerly accepted the diploma from the president of the college, Milton Eisenhower. In fact, I grabbed it from his hand before he could change his mind and withdraw it. I might soon be working for Milton's brother, Ike, but that night the handshake and words of congratulations from Milton meant more to me than any future honor I could foresee.

The Army Needs Warm Bodies

VETERINARIANS have a choice of fields to enter upon graduation. Originally I had planned to enter government service because of the security it offered. World War II changed the the plans of most who were graduating during those years. The members of the classes graduating before my class were called into service immediately upon graduation. Although the cavalry had been disbanded, veterinarians were needed in food inspection and other health activities. By the time my class graduated in 1944, the veterinary corps had obtained sufficient personnel. Only a few in my class were called into service. The rest of us were thrown back on the mercy of our local draft boards. If you were under twenty-six and physically fit, your chances for induction were excellent, even though a veterinary advisory board did try to protect veterinary practitioners who were in livestock areas that were critically short on veterinarians. Since my father had conducted his practice by himself up until that date, there was little reason for me to expect a deferment by returning to work with him. Government service would not protect a person. However, as I had originally planned to enter that service, I took employment with the Meat Inspection Service while awaiting the call of my draft board.

The draft boards were hungry for bodies to fill quotas. My father and my grandfather before him had served in our country's armed forces. I had no objection to serving; I just didn't want to squander my education by serving as a buck private. I contacted the army, the navy, the marine corps, the coast guard, the maritime service, and any other entity I heard of to see if they would accept me in their medical corps. I was under twenty-six. They had orders to keep their hands off persons like myself. The draft boards needed warm bodies.

The dilemma I faced was self-created. I had only to acknowledge that I had suffered an attack of rheumatic fever and I would have been declared 4F (physically unqualified). My whole future would have been changed. Any person who was physically fit and 4F in those days had his pick of jobs. I was too stupid or too proud to admit to having a physical defect. After all, no physical exam could detect any abnormalities. I had spent one summer hitchhiking and sleeping out and the next summer working on a paving crew during the day and carousing at night without a relapse. I wasn't going to have a relapse! I never acknowledged to any examining doctor or on any medical history report that I had ever suffered from rheumatic fever. I wasn't trying to be heroic by refusing to hide behind an "imaginary disability." I just didn't want to be considered a coward.

That summer Marian and I moved to St. Louis where I went to work inspecting meat for the U.S. Meat Inspection Service. (Marian got a job working in an office at a war plant.) I had originally planned to enter government service upon graduation; however, meat inspection was an entirely different field than any I had been exposed to before that time. I probably wouldn't have stayed with it even if the war hadn't upset my plans. The work was repetitious and the environment was a far cry from the out-of-doors of a rural veterinary practice or the indoors of a modern veterinary hospital.

Most of us eat meat. We realize that the animals have to be killed, and most have at least a vague conception that the meat is inspected by veterinarians before it is passed for food. Most, however, have no idea of the procedures involved. Although this period occupied but a brief time in my life, a few remarks may be in order.

Animals were driven into the killing pens connected with the processing floors. In this case a different species was processed on each floor; thus hogs, cattle, and sheep and goats were handled on different floors. Cattle were stunned with a sledge hammer blow to the head, suspended by their hind legs from an overhead moving chain, and bled out by having their jugular vein cut. Swine were suspended fully conscious to have their jugulars severed by a knife. The killers worked in the killing pits hour after hour. How the men's sanity, let alone their ears, survived the screaming of the dying hogs is still a wonder to me. Since those days, however, they have developed humane methods to make the animals unconscious before proceeding with the slaughter.

Antemortem inspections were conducted before the animals were driven to the slaughter floors to eliminate obviously sick animals from being killed for food. The slaughtered and bled-out animals were then skinned out in the case of the cattle and sheep or goats or dehaired in the case of the hogs. The next procedure was to eviscerate the animals by making a midline incision with a knife and cleaver, tying off the bung (the anal opening of the intestine), and dropping the intact viscera into a pan by cutting the tissues suspending the viscera from the dorsal body wall and from the neck area. The veterinarian or lay inspector would then inspect the viscera for lesions of disease. This procedure was carried out visually and by the incision of certain glands and tissues. Because much of the process was done or accompanied by the manipulation of the viscera with bare hands, the process became known as "gut puddling," and the inspectors involved in those activities were known as "gut puddlers."

Cattle only moved by us at the rate of twenty to thirty an hour, so one person could easily handle the necessary inspection work. Hogs moved by at the rate of up to six hundred an hour. The process of removing hair from the hogs was far faster than that of skinning out the cattle. One inspector was supposed to be able to handle a hog line if not running over three hundred an hour as long as he got periodic rest breaks. When over that speed, two inspectors were used. The inspector had the choices of passing the carcass for food, holding it in an examination room for further and final inspection by the "final" inspector, or condemning the carcass. A stamp was available to stamp the condemned viscera and carcasses. A set of numbered tags was used to identify the suspicious viscera and the corresponding carcass hanging in back of it. When stamped or tagged, carcasses and viscera passed down the chain line and pan line to the area of the "final room"; here they were shuttled off the main line and into that area for action by the final inspector. Needless to say, a person working on a line with a carcass and viscera passing his station every few seconds had to be constantly alert. The experienced inspectors handled the work without difficulty. Neophytes, like myself, worked under the tutelage of experienced personnel while we were learning the "art and science of puddling guts."

Another problem that went with the job was that of skin rash on the hands. After working on the cattle floor for a few days, I developed the cattle itch. Both hands were red and had a rash all over them. About the time I had finally overcome this affliction, I was transferred to the hog floor, and after a few days I developed the hog itch. We were transferred from floor to floor monthly. The itch was due to the temperature of the viscera which we were examining with our bare hands. Each species had a different temperature and thus the cattle itch, hog itch, and the like developed. The skin eventually developed a tolerance for the temperatures contacted and the rashes did not occur. However, the time involved in developing this tolerance was more than the time I spent there.

Cadavers that were condemned were cut up in the "final room" and dropped down an enclosed stainless steel chute into a condemned room. Within this room an employee cut up the cadaver or parts further and handled the necessary incineration, processing for fertilizer, and so forth. This employee would be locked in the room every morning with his lunch. At the end of the day, the room would be unlocked and he was released. One day a newcomer to the job was heard pounding on the inside of the door. When they looked through the window, they saw a man, white as a sheet, pounding on the door and urgently signaling to be released. When they opened the door, he fled, never to be seen again. To me, this job would have been far better than that of killing hogs, but every man to his own tastes.

In the meantime, my draft board kept track of my whereabouts and kept a stream of correspondence coming my way. They finally moved me into the slot for a preinduction physical. I was issued a summons to take a trip to nearby Jefferson Barracks to take the physical. Upon arrival at Jefferson Barracks, I joined long lines of boys and men being processed through the medical center. Boys might not be old enough to vote, to buy liquor, to get married until they were twenty-one, but they were old enough to fight and die at eighteen. The army needed soldiers.

The medics took my temperature and pulse. They peered into my mouth, my eyes, and my ears. I removed my clothes on command and they looked me over just like a horse buyer would look over a stud before buying.

"Turn around. Bend over. Spread your cheeks. No, your butt, Junior. O.K. Stand up and move on."

"O.K. Turn your head and cough," he ordered. A medic was seated in front of me and held a surgically gloved hand up in my inguinal area. He moved his hand to the other side. "Turn your head the other way and cough again." He took a disdainful look at my genitals and turned his head away. Embarrassed, I looked down. Everything seemed normal to me. The medic in front of me was probably a disillusioned surgeon who, like myself, was involved in activities he felt below his training.

"Put your arm flat on the table. Make a fist. Hold it. Steady. That's it. Hold the cotton over the vein. Move on. Next." He methodically passed the vial of blood to an aide who wrote down the pertinent identification information on the label.

"Take this bottle into the next room and fill it with urine."

The young boy ahead of me in the next room looked down and

sprawled on the floor in a dead faint. He looked pale. Probably that medic had been overly enthusiastic when he drew blood from him.

"Get back! Give him air!"

"Give the boy air!"

A whiff of smelling salts caused him to open his eyes. In a few minutes he was up.

"Here's your bottle. Fill it up." The boy voided and moved on to the next room. The army needed warm bodies. Fainting wasn't cause for rejection.

Finally, we were allowed to put our clothes back on and regain some of our dignity. Then came the medical history reports. Again I failed to mention that I had had rheumatic fever. The physical was passed with flying colors. I awaited my induction notice.

One evening, a short time before I was to report for induction, Marian and I were attending a movie. The movie was interrupted to flash a notice on the screen. The U.S. Maritime Service was now accepting persons for training. It was desperately in need of personnel to man the liberty ships that the shipbuilders were assembling in ever-increasing numbers. The ships were needed to supply our troops around the globe. Trained sailors were not available in sufficient numbers to man the growing fleet. The maritime service had been granted dispensation to accept able-bodied persons under twenty-six years of age. The next day I signed up with the maritime service to take hospital corps-purser training. Each ship was a self-contained unit. The person who took care of the books was also responsible for any medical treatment that the crew might require. I felt I was better qualified than most and would get to use my training to some extent so was happy.

A group of fellow enlistees from the southern Missouri and northern Arkansas area joined me on a coach car of the Baltimore and Ohio Railroad and were given a free trip to the training camp at Sheepshead Bay, New York. Sheepshead Bay was located on Long Island just east of Brooklyn. Most of the fellow enlistees were, like myself, trying to beat the draft. Most of them, unlike myself, were only eighteen years of age and had seldom been away from the small villages and rural areas of the Ozarks. Spending weekends in New York City was to be an experience for them. Our group was combined to form a unit with a group of fishermen of Portugese extraction from Gloucester, Massachusetts. They said they were from "Glowster." It took me several days to learn that they meant Gloucester. My colleagues said they came from "Arkansaw" but everybody knew they meant Arkansas. To say you were from Glowster was confusing to a middlewesterner.

After arrival we were again stripped of our dignity. First we exchanged the civilian clothes we arrived in for navy gear. I was fitted out in bell-bottom trousers, jackets, peacoat—the whole works. From outward appearances we were sailors. Inwardly, I had a lot to learn. I still have my dress uniform stored in a trunk. How I ever managed to get into those trousers is a mystery. I must have been 100 pounds lighter and used talc powder on my hips for lubrication.

One of the first things we learned was that which was taught in all branches of the services—namely, hurry up and wait. We stood in line for roll call, for duty assignments, for chow; you name it, we stood in line for it. For several years after I got out of the service I refused to stand in line for anything. It took time for me to disassociate standing in line with a degrading experience.

Initially, we all went through the same introductory training. After that we were given advanced training in the field for which we were selected. During the initial training we moved as a unit. Each unit had a leader and an assistant leader who had charge of the group and marched them from one place to another or directed them in parade-ground drill. I can possibly understand the necessity of marching the unit from one classroom to the other; I cannot understand the necessity of teaching close-order drill. It was certainly never used on the liberty ships. Anyway, another fellow from St. Louis and myself were the only ones who had ever had military training. I had taken ROTC in college. We were the only ones who knew the difference between right face and left dress so that qualified us to be the leaders. The only advantage I received from it was an extra weekend night to spend with Marian.

After I was shipped out of St. Louis, Marian went to Miami to visit her parents. After I finished my fourteen-day quarantine, she came to New York and got a job on Wall Street to be near me. She found an apartment in Brooklyn and we used this as a weekend home. The network of subways covered the New York metropolitan area even to the gates of Sheepshead Bay, so traveling back and forth was no problem. We did get an opportunity to see New York City. We took in shows, sporting events, the parks and, on occasion, the bars on Saturday nights.

The bars were restricted to persons twenty-one years and over. I was twenty-one, but most of my fellow trainees were not. They did have access to the Pepsi Cola Canteen sponsored by the USO; however, to a person under twenty-one, the restriction on purchasing alcoholic beverages often seemed unfair. A group of us adults would sit at a table near the window at the Brass Rail and wave to our adolescent colleagues who had their noses pressed against the window. This was something far different from the night life in "Farmville" where they came from.

I was told that the ladies' room of the Brass Rail had a male figurine, nude except for a projecting fig leaf that covered its genital area. The leaf was hinged and attached to a concealed bell that rang loudly throughout the establishment whenever someone lifted the leaf to see what might be underneath. Whenever an unsuspecting lady entered the powder room, an expectant silence would fall on the regular clientele. If the bell rang in a few minutes, an uproarious guffaw would greet the embarrassed and red-faced lady as she came back out from the powder room.

"What happened to you in there?"

"You know what happened."

"No, I don't. I'm a gentleman and can't go in there."

"You're no gentleman or you wouldn't laugh."

"Well, maybe you're no lady or you wouldn't have tried to rob Adam of his dignity."

On Saturday mornings before we left on leaves we lined up as usual. This time it was for a genital inspection.

Woe be to the man who had a drop of mucous appear at his urethral orifice. He was restricted and sent to sick bay to be started on sulfa tablets. Whether this reduced the amount of VD in New York is doubtful. Since gonorrhea is painful to the man and there was no stigma attached to seeking treatment, probably few additional cases were found. Even if the available female population had been checked, it might not have reduced the VD rate. Many years later in public health school, a doctor who served with the U.S. Army told me of his experiences in running regular checks for the U.S. Army on the ladies at the red-light houses in Naples, Italy. He didn't believe it reduced the VD rate one iota. Further, he said, if he ever had had any desires to patronize such houses in the past, they were certainly dissipated after having to make the necessary physical examinations on the professionals.

Part of the training activities involved learning to row boats around the bay. By this time it was getting cold; zero weather and freezing rain were common. We dressed in slickers, rubber hats, and gloves, but we still got wet to the skin and chilled to the bone. There was no relief from the cold in an open whaleboat. The surf was rough, although I'm certain the administration didn't send us out in the boats when the surf was too rough. They thought too much of their boats to do that. I don't know if I would have survived if I had had to abandon ship on the North Atlantic after a German U-Boat attack. The thing that may have saved us at Sheepshead Bay was the presence of the Portugese fishermen in our group. They took to the boats like veterans. Whatever boatsmanship I learned, I owe to these colleagues.

When the basic training was completed, I entered the hospital corps training. It was a twelve-week course with examinations given every two weeks. Since it was elementary material for me, I arranged to take the course in six weeks. Every week I would move up to the class ahead of me and take the exam with them. If I passed, I could do the same the next week.

I had no trouble and was halfway through the training program when I began to get a stiffness in my back. It was particularly severe when I arose in the morning but after moving around, it would ameliorate so that I could get through the day without difficulty. I thought nothing about it. I spent that weekend as usual with Marian. My back was bothering me, but I wasn't going to let that slow me down—especially on my weekend leave. The next week my back kept getting worse but I refused to check into sick bay. That weekend I lay around during the days at the apartment. On Saturday night we went to Madison Square Garden to see a basketball game but Sunday night I wasn't up to leaving the apartment. Monday morning I managed to limp back into the base and headed for sick bay. I didn't know what was wrong with me but I knew I was sick.

Sick bays are managed by technicians with only superficial medical training. They were unfamiliar with illnesses like mine. As far as they knew I might only be trying to "gold brick." I lay in a cot in sick bay for a couple of days without my back improving and receiving very little attention. On the third day my knee began to throb and swell painfully. I knew then what was wrong. After four years, I was having a rheumatic fever relapse. I told the medics what was wrong and requested transfer to the hospital where I could receive proper care. At first they ignored me. Finally, the next night, I figured I had better do something drastic or they were going to leave me there untreated until too late to protect my health. Accordingly, I moaned off and on all night long, which wasn't hard to do because of the way I felt. It got results. The medics didn't like to have their sick bay disturbed by someone moaning, so they saw that I was transferred to the hospital the next day.

I was quartered in the hospital with a group of other persons suffering from rheumatic fever. Some, like myself, were suffering from relapses. They, too, had lied about previous attacks in order to gain admission into the service. Unless a person is unfortunate enough to suffer valvular heart damage, it is impossible during a physical examination to tell that he has had a previous attack. The maritime service was not happy with the lot of us who had falsified our records. They had been out considerable expense training us and now were out the expense of treating us until we were back on our feet and could be released. From our standpoint it also was not a pleasant situation. The U.S. Maritime Service is not one of the armed services. It was a training program for commercial work. Consequently, when we received a medical discharge from the maritime service, we were not entitled to any disability payments. This left us in a defenseless position. The penalty for our actions of falsifying papers was paid several times over. The maritime service was unhappy, Marian was unhappy, and I was unhappy.

I lay in the hospital bed looking out the window at the ship convoys entering and leaving New York harbor. I was regaled with stories of the German U-Boats lying just off the mouth of the harbor during the early months of the war. They sank our ships as they emerged from the harbor, their silhouettes outlined against the skyline of New York. We were told of newly graduated trainees taking their first boat out of New York on ships that were sunk. The boys ended up in the hospital with badly burned bodies less than twenty-four hours after finishing training. The war was real to Sheepshead Bay in those early war years. Few ships were being sunk by the time I landed in the hospital. I lay in the bed counting the ships as they appeared over the horizon to enter the harbor or as they emerged one by one from the harbor to form convoys for the journey across the North Atlantic.

My service was over, the days passed slowly, and I had to find a job. I believed in rheumatic fever relapses now. After discussions with my physician, I decided that I had better take a regular-hour job rather than enter a large animal practice like my father had conducted. The exposure to meat inspection had been enough. I wanted something different. For a short time I forgot my phobia about classrooms. I answered an advertisement in the *Journal of the American Veterinary Medical Association* for a position in the Department of Veterinary Medicine at Purdue University and was accepted. Since I was making a good recovery, my physician discharged me early so I could arrive at Lafayette, Indiana, by the required date.

I had a hassle with the maritime service before I left. I was being thrown out on the street without a pension. Beyond that they wanted to strip me of my service wardrobe and throw me out on the streets practically in my underclothes. I protested the impropriety of walking the streets of New York in that attire. I had no extra money. My pay had been only twenty-one dollars a month, hardly enough to take care of beer money and subway fares. After some lengthy quibbling, they rescinded that order and were going to discharge me with my dress blues and nothing more. Again we argued. It was below zero outside. My heavy clothes were in Fredonia, Kansas. I needed the peacoat.

"That's your problem. It's government property."

"It's your problem if I get sick because I'll write my congressman. I'm not leaving here without the peacoat."

"The hell you aren't. Give me the coat and get out."

"See this chair. I'm sitting here until you agree to let me have this peacoat. It's cold out there."

My stubborness finally convinced them that I was serious. I was allowed to leave with the peacoat. I'm certain Uncle Sam never missed the coat. I'm sure I would have frozen without it.

I spent the few intervening days before our scheduled departure at the apartment. Although I didn't exert myself, I did some sightseeing. The night before were were to leave we had dinner at the apartment of one of Marian's fellow workers. The lady lived on the New Jersey side of the Hudson River and there was a beautiful view of the New York skyline—even though it was dim-out conditions. Life was beginning to look wonderful. I was looking forward to returning to the college campus again. I may have had an extra drink or two to celebrate the event. Anyway, I finally went to sleep late that night back at our Brooklyn apartment content with the world.

The next morning I awoke to find my left knee swollen to twice its normal size.

"Marian, I don't think I can move. My knee is swollen."

"Can you go back to the hospital?"

"No. They discharged me and don't want to see me again."

"Well, I quit my job and I certainly don't want to stay in New York any longer."

"They won't take me at Purdue in this condition."

"Then let's get a train to Miami. If I'm going to have to work and take care of you too, let's do it in Miami where my parents are."

I wasn't in a position to argue the point. Marian arranged by telephone to transfer the train tickets from Lafayette to Miami. She then went out and purchased some crutches for me. Later that day, when everything was arranged, she telephoned for a taxi. Somehow the cab driver and Marian managed to get me down the stairs into the cab and out of the cab and into the train station. Marian got me onto the train and into my seat. My future, which looked so bright twenty-four hours earlier, now looked dismal.

Marian's parents met us at the Miami station and took us to their Coral Gables home. I now knew how to take care of myself. No need to see a doctor. Rest, sulfa, and lots of aspirin tablets would do the trick. Marian went out and got a job. I basked in the sun and swallowed tablets in huge quantities. Whether it was the sun, the rest, the aspirins, or all three—I don't know. However the swelling receded, the aches and pains disappeared, and I started moving around without my crutches.

Just when I felt my troubles might be behind me, I received another notice from my draft board. They were still short on men so I was ordered to take another of those free trips with a group of potential inductees, this time to Camp Blanding, Florida, to take a physical. Again I went through the physical. By now I was learning when to bend over, when to make a fist, and when to turn my head and cough without being told. Again the doctors could find nothing wrong with me.

"Doctor, you can take me but I have had rheumatic fever." This time I told the truth.

"Let me listen to your heart again."

"You won't hear anything."

"What proof do I have that you've had rheumatic fever? How do I know that you aren't just trying to avoid serving your country?"

"Well, I got discharged from the maritime service at Sheepshead Bay four months ago."

"You've got to be kidding."

"No, I'm not. You can contact them for documentation." I gave him the pertinent information.

For one week I was boarded at the army's expense before confirmation was received from the maritime service. I returned to Miami with mixed emotions and a 4F card. I was free at last. The question was, what was I capable of doing?

Although I visited some of the few veterinarians in Miami at that time, I was not then interested in small animal practice. I had been raised in a cattle and hog practice with a different type of clientele. I presumed it would be difficult to get a job with an institution or with the government with my history of rheumatic fever relapses. I remembered having to turn down the appointment to Purdue. I began to think of returning to Fredonia, Kansas, to work with my father. He was advancing in years. The Depression was over, and the life was more financially rewarding than when I was growing up. Besides, with two veterinarians working in the practice, I would be able to take it easy if my aches and pains came back. After consultation with my father, it was agreed that I should return to work with him. Thus I prepared to embark upon the first lengthy part of my professional career.

We moved back to Fredonia and stayed temporarily with my parents until we could find a place of our own. Dad bought me a used car and provided me with some medicines and necessary equipment so I was ready to start practicing. Marian took charge of answering the telephone calls and people coming to the door. My mother decided to pursue a teaching career since she was no longer tied to the telephone. Marian soon learned what a "fresh" cow was, how to get specific directions to the farms, and what the "male" animal was. The farm ladies never used the word "bull" for some reason or other, thinking it was a dirty word. She often joined me in the evenings, riding along to take care of evening calls. She would visit the ladies at the house while I went to the barn with the farmer. Sometimes she observed the barnyard surgery or treatment and that way learned something about livestock. For a city girl, it was quite a startling change of life. She adapted well, though, for we stayed there for about fifteen years, except for the sixteen months we were in Mexico.*

---

*This experience related in a previous book, *Doctor, Spare My Cow.* Iowa State College Press, Ames, Iowa. 1956.

"Can Junior Vet?"

"Can he vet?"
"He's a graduate veterinarian."
"Yes, but can he vet?"
"Of course he can vet."
"Armer isn't there, you say?"
"No, Armer isn't here but his son is."
"Well, send Junior out then."

When I first started out practicing I did have to learn to vet. When riding with my father in former years I had paid little attention to the diagnosing and treatment of diseases. At Kansas State College we were confronted by the esoteric rather than the usual run-of-the-mill sick animal cases. If the case was normal, the local veterinarian would handle it. If it was a problem, he might send it to the college to get it and the owner out of his hair.

At college I learned of the seven cases reported in the literature of herniation of the omentum of the cow through the left inguinal canal, the thirteen cases reported of the rupture of the prepubic tendon, and the like. In practice, I had to learn to diagnose the more common ailments such as impaction, pneumonia, and hardware.

Furthermore, I had to learn materia medica from an applied point of view. During the twenty years intervening between the time my father started practicing and when I started, the medicines used had changed very little. Now 80 percent of the drugs we are using will be replaced by other drugs within ten years. That is, this condition was true until recently. Now stricter restrictions on the licensing of new drugs is slowing this turnover down considerably. However, when I started out I could get by with a couple of dozen different medicines in my practice car. My father did insist that I know the toxic dose of the drugs used.

As he so aptly put it, "If you don't kill them, most of them will get well."

Today we do have miracle drugs that at least partially outdate this statement.

Marian also had to learn. She was from the city and knew little of the farm. She had to learn to converse in a new language.

"Is Doc there?"

"No, can I help you?"

"Not unless you're a vet. Is Armer around?"

"No, but I expect my husband back within the hour. Can I give him a message?"

"Yes. Tell him to get out here as soon as he can. I have a cow that freshened. She's down and looks like she is dying."

"You say she freshened?"

"Yes. F-R-E-S-H-E-N-E-D. Freshened. Get him out here fast."

"I'm sorry this isn't Sybil. I'm Dr. Porter, Jr.'s, wife. I don't recognize your voice. To whom am I speaking?" All the time Marian was wondering what freshened referred to.

"Hell, Mrs. Porter, I thought everybody knew my voice. This is Bert McGee."

"Hello, Mr. McGee. I'll try to recognize your voice next time. Does my husband know where you live?" She was wondering if she should ask what freshening meant or would I know.

"Sure, he's been here plenty of times with Armer."

"Well, maybe you'd better tell me. He may have forgotten." If she asked what freshened meant, he'd just think she was stupid. She would wait and ask me when I came in. I would know.

"Just tell him to come to the old Summer place out west of town. Tell him to go across the river at Smith's Ford and then take the left fork for two miles. My farm is the one on the left with the house with the red roof."

"All right, Mr. McGee. I'll send my husband out as soon as he arrives."

"You come along and meet the missus. You need to learn where the McGee's place is at. Besides Betty Ann hasn't had any company all week. She'll talk your ears off."

Marian's curiosity was aroused. What in the world was a fresh cow. Did it act "fresh" around other cows or the owner? Well, she would ask me when I came in.

When I arrived she transferred the office calls over to Sybil at the other house and jumped into the car with me. She was going to find out what a fresh cow was.

"Well, a fresh cow is one that has just had a calf. Fresh means that she has just come to her milk."

"Why don't they just say she had a calf? Freshened sounds peculiar." She later learned to accept that terminology as proper along with the words "cleaned" for removal of a retained placenta (afterbirth), "impacted" for constipation, "heaves" for heavy breathing, and others that slip my mind now.

When we arrived, Bert directed me to the barnyard where a cow was lying on her side completely unaware of the world around her. A quick glance informed me she was still breathing.

"Bert, roll this cow up on her stomach or she's going to be dead in a few minutes and then you'll say I killed her."

I grabbed a nose lead and inserted it into the cow's nostrils so that her head could be held in a fixed position around on her side while I administered a bottle of calcium solution intravenously into her jugular vein.

"Doc, you know that Sam Brooks calls you 'Doc-Kill-Em-Quick'?"

"Well, his cow was breathing her last when I started giving the medicine. She had pneumonia. I should have arrived a few minutes later so she'd been dead before I started giving the medicine or I should have been called two days earlier while I could still do some good."

The cow was beginning to breathe more regularly. Betty Ann had arrived to take Marian in tow.

"I'm Betty Ann, Bert's wife. Don't pay any attention to Bert. He's just nervous about Blue. She is our best milk cow. Bert was offered $225 for her and wouldn't like to lose her."

"If she gets up, I'm going to sell her the next time I get that good an offer."

"Don't do it, Bert," I said. "Only good cows have milk fever. Why up at the Fredonia Dairy they're eager to buy cows that have had this condition, which we call milk fever. Milk fever is a sign they give lots of milk."

"Milk fever is a sign of a veterinary bill. Maybe you don't charge Jack up at the Dairy as much because he's close to your office."

"Well, that is right, but this cow is still worth my veterinary fee."

"I'll have to see if she lives and what you charge before I can answer that."

Betty Ann was leading Marian away. "Bert is just a born pessimist."

Blue's eyes began to roll around in their sockets. She stretched her hind legs and tried to pull her head loose from the nose lead.

"Hold onto that nose lead, Bert. Blue is beginning to wake up. She needs this whole bottle before you let her loose."

"If Blue lives I'll tell Sam Brooks that I'm going to call you 'Doctor-Bring-Em-Back-to-Life.'"

"Blue's going to live."

Blue mooed and attempted to get her head loose from the nose restraint. A calf lying nearby bawled. It arose and staggered over to Blue.

"It's a bull calf," said Bert. "That's the sign of a poor farmer; bull calves and girl babies, and I have my share of both."

I had finished the IV administration of the calcium.

"Bert, take the nose lead out of her nose and let her look around."

By the time I had cleaned up my equipment and put it away, Blue had staggered to her feet. The calf was soon nosing around her flank searching for a teat to suckle on.

"Doc, I told you I'm going to tell Sam Brooks that your name is 'Doctor-Bring-Em-Back-To-Life.' I would have sold Blue cheap thirty minutes ago. How much do I owe you for the resurrection?"

"I guess ten dollars ought to do it."

"I'll go up to the house and get the check book. I think I saw the women folk heading out for the cider press. You'd better go out and see what they're doing."

I found Betty and Marian out at the cider press. It was under an open shed. Behind was an entrance to a cellar.

"Bert keeps the cider down there so it can age and keep cool."

Betty explained the process of expressing the juice from the apples and converting it into cider. Bert rejoined us and handed me a check.

"Here's your check, Doc. You earned it today. I've got something special you need to sample before you go." He went down the steps into the cellar and returned within a few minutes with a jug.

"Let's go up to the house and get some glasses."

We walked up to the house and entered Betty Ann's immaculately clean kitchen. A wooden cookstove was on one side of the room, a sink with a hand pump on the other. On the other two sides were cupboards whose open shelves revealed a beautiful array of china and the so-called china and crystal antiques. In the center of the room was a table covered with a checkered oilcloth and four chairs.

"Pull up chairs, you two. Betty Ann, get some glasses out. You two are going to be treated to McGee's special stock."

Bert pulled the corncob stopper from the jug and filled the four glasses. Betty Ann put a glass in front of each of us and she and Bert pulled up chairs and joined us.

"Now, Marian, go easy on that," Betty Ann was advising.

We raised our glasses in a toast and then took a swallow. Marian coughed sharply and hurriedly put her glass down. I felt a warm burning sensation descending my esophagus as the liquid moved down.

"Bert should have warned you. He put a little extra fermenting material in that special jug and it hasn't aged enough yet. It still is a little raw on the gizzard." She took a swallow. "What do you think, Bert, three more months?"

Bert was finishing his glass and urging me along. "No more than three months, Betty Ann. I think it'll be as good as the batch we made in '36." He turned his attention to me. "That's going to be some real hard cider. Nobody outside of the McGees knows the recipe. It's been handed down from generation to generation ever since the McGees left the Old Country." He was refilling my glass.

Before I knew it I had downed three glasses, matching Bert glass for glass. Marian was still sipping on her first glass and warily watching me.

"Doc, were you in the service?"

Before I could reply, Bert launched into stories about his service in Company E of the local National Guard. It had served overseas during World War I.

"I served under your father, Armer. He was first sergeant. He was real efficient, but he couldn't pronounce some words. I remember he couldn't pronounce 'l.' He would say brue for blue and brouse for blouse." Bert soon got carried away reminiscing about his war experiences. I had never heard my father say much about his service years so I listened. We matched glass for glass. Bert became more talkative and I became more light-headed. Marian became more apprehensive.

Finally, after several glasses too many, Marian began to hint that we had to get home. Bert urged her to take one more sip. "Doc needs a rest. Besides he's never had real hard cider before. Armer can cover the calls tonight."

By that time Bert and I were raising toasts to the victory of the Argonne Forest, to Company E, to Armistice Day, to VJ Day, to VE Day; you name it, we toasted it.

Marian finally rolled me into the car and drove home.

"Now you know what a fresh cow is," I said sleepily.

"Yes, and I know what a drunken ex-sailor looks like. You'd better stay away from hard cider in the future."

"But Bert wanted me to taste it. I had to be sociable."

"I thought you were going to drop her beautiful glass when you drank that toast to VJ Day. They'll probably think you're a drunk and never have you again."

I didn't answer her; I had nearly passed out. I muttered, "Doctor-Bring-Em-Back-Alive. Not bad."

"What did you say?"

I was asleep. I slumped in the seat with a big grin on my face. Marian looked over at me and frowned.

"I wonder what girl he's dreaming about now?"

The Old Maids' Sick Hog

BELLE and Marge Dawson were two old-maid sisters who farmed eighty acres out north of town. Although my father had done work for them over the years, I had neither been on their farm nor personally met them until my return to Fredonia as a practicing veterinarian. I had, however, often seen them in their fields or around their yard as I drove by. They still farmed with a team of horses. Their neighbors said they could harness a team as well as any man. In warm weather they wore long-sleeved dresses with skirts that came below their knees, high-top work shoes with long socks, and straw or felt hats. In the winter or in inclement weather they wore long cloth overcoats and rubber boots or high-buckle overshoes. Both were as thin as a rail with faces well weathered and creased from exposure to the elements.

On Saturdays they would drive their Model T into town and park in front of the produce store to sell their cream and eggs. They would probably have preferred to be driving their horse and buggy to town, but the hitching posts had been taken down about thirty years before and the cars would have spooked the horse. Anyway, they had acquired a Model T car in which to make this weekly trip. They would take the proceeds from the sale of their produce and go to the grocery store to buy the flour, sugar, and other staples they would need for the coming week. In those days the cream and egg money kept the necessary staples in the cupboard. The intermediate processors did a minimum amount of repackaging or reprocessing and consequently claimed a minimum amount of the grocery dollar. Five dollars would buy several sacks of groceries. When they had completed their shopping, Belle would climb up into the Model T and seat herself behind the steering wheel while Marge went around to the front to "man" the crank. When Belle had the spark and gas levers adjusted, Marge would raise her skirt up above her knees and step over and straddle the front bumper. Astraddle the bumper she would then take hold of the crank, position the crank and herself, look up at Belle to see if she was ready, then give the crank a couple of strong turns. The engine would cough and then sputter into life. Marge extricated herself from the position astraddle the bumper, smoothed the wrinkles out of her go-to-town dress, walked around the side of the car opposite the driver, and climbed up into the seat. Belle would then back away from the curb, put the car in forward gear, and the two would head for home.

One day my mother relayed a call to me from the old-maid Dawsons. They had a sick hog, Armer wasn't going to be back for several hours, and they wanted somebody right away. They would try Junior.

I drove into their yard and was directed to a pen out near their barn. The pen was about fifteen feet by fifteen feet. The fence was woven wire about three feet high supported on some wooden posts that looked like they were ready to collapse at any time. A shed was located in one corner of the pen; it was roofed and enclosed on three sides by metal corrugated sheets with the side facing Belle and me being open. The roof was about four feet high. Looking across into the shadows of the shed I saw a large hog. Its eyes were riveted on me. The pen was a wallow. I didn't see a dry place outside the shed. Most of the pen looked like it was six inches deep in a stinking blend of hog manure, rain water, and mud. A feed trough was resting just inside the fence. It was supported on tiles to keep it from being submerged in the mire.

The situation did not look inviting. How in the world had my father managed to treat animals under these conditions? There was no place that the hog could be confined for an examination and I dreaded the thought of climbing into the pen. The stench was bad enough standing outside.

"What seems to be wrong with the hog?" I cautiously inquired.

"I wouldn't have called you out if I knew," Belle rebuffed me.

I saw that this wasn't going to be easy. "Can you tell me how long he has been sick?"

"He hasn't eaten his slop for three days."

I look in the trough. It was half full of a stinking mess that she called slop. If I had been the hog, I wouldn't have eaten it either. I looked over towards the shelter. The hog lay there with its eyes watching my every move. It might or might not be sick; however, it was obvious it had no intention of missing any of my actions. Men seldom came on the farm. What was I up to?

"Did you try changing feed?"

"No. Why? Hogs always eat slop."

"Just what is in your slop?"

"Shorts, table scraps, and dish water. Just what is always in slop,"

Belle replied testily. It was obvious to her that she should have waited for Armer. Junior didn't know anything about slop.

"Well, maybe the hog needs a change of feed. His eyes look alert to me. Why don't you get a couple of ears of corn?"

With a look of disgust and resignation she went out to the barn and opened the door to the feed bin to get the corn. She knew by now this was going to be a waste of her money. I didn't know anything about hogs.

"Aren't you going to take its temperature?" As long as she was going to have to pay a veterinary bill she might as well get her money's worth.

The situation was looking more hopeless by the minute. How was I going to confine the hog to make any type of examiniation, let alone treat it?

"Armer would take the hog's temperature." She was waiting for me to get into that pen with her hog. It smelled bad enough outside. I didn't want to climb inside.

"Have you got a piece of baling wire?" She wasn't going to allow me to leave without performing like a vet.

When she returned with the wire, I passed the free end of the wire through the end with the loop. After adjustment I had a noose at one end that I might, with luck, be able to slip into the hog's mouth and secure back of its tusks. I wrapped the free end around my palm and straightened the wire noose out. I had seen my father do this on many occasions. I had never used this method, but I was being forced to try it.

I leaned over the fence and waved one of the ears of corn at the hog. When I had its attention. I dropped the ear in the feed trough and stood erect. I still held the wire noose in postion near the trough. Would the hog take the bait? The hog slowly arose and sniffed the air a few times.

"Pig! Pig! Pig!" I cautiously tried to coax the hog out of the shed. The hog just stood there.

Maid Belle shook her head. "Here, let me show you how to do this." She reached down and picked up a club lying nearby. Leaning over the fence, she beat on the side of the trough with the club, uttering a cry as if the pig was in the next county. "Sueeeey, here pig! Pig! Pig! Sueeeey. Sueeeey. Sueeeey." The pig started out of the shed into the wallow. Its first step found it sinking up to its belly in the grime. If I had been the hog I wouldn't have waded through the filth to eat either. The Old Maid Belle had a satisfied look on her face. She had shown up the kid.

"See, you just have to know how to talk to a pig."

"Miss Dawson, I can see that you know how."

The hog slowly half-waded, half-swam across the wallow. When it reached the trough, it used its front feet to hoist its front end up out of the slime and into the trough. He smelled the ear of corn gingerly. I desperately tried to work the wire noose into its mouth while it started chewing the ear. Just when I about succeeded, he dislodged the noose with a shake of his head. Again I tried, and again he thwarted my efforts. Finally, when it was beginning to look hopeless, I succeeded and quickly pulled the noose tight back of his tusks. The startled hog gave a shrill shriek and jumped back, pulling the wire out of my hand. Luckily it didn't cut my palm but I was faced with a loose hog and an irate owner.

"Now look what you've done. Armer wouldn't have let him get away."

I grunted. This was getting more disgusting by the minute. "I think your hog will be all right. He ate the corn. Why don't we leave him be and you call me tomorrow if he's not all right?"

"Son, you don't leave here until you examine that hog. It is sick. You can at least take its temperature." She was adamant. I wasn't going to get away that easy.

"I'm sorry I don't know how we'll catch the hog now. It's going to be real spooky."

"It's got a noose in its snout, hasn't it? Get in there and catch it. This time hold on to it until you get it wrapped someplace."

I looked at Belle Dawson. She meant it. I looked at the wallow. Why did I have to get caught with this call?

"Young man, get in there and doctor that hog. Armer would."

I shook my head in disbelief. Obviously she wasn't going to let me leave that easily. Gingerly I stepped over the fence into the mire. I sank nearly to the top of my rubber boots. The aroma rose around me. The hog warily watched my movements from the far corner of the pen.

I moved towards it. It swam and waded quickly out of reach. I looked over at Belle. She was staring impassively at me. Her face betrayed no sympathy. I looked back at the hog and moved towards its new location. Again it quickly evaded me. I tried again. This time the hog darted near me. I grabbed for and caught the wire. The hog was pulled up short. I looked around rapidly for a place to anchor the snare. The hog took advantage of the diversion of my attention, made a turn and swam the other way. I was caught off balance and fell on my backside in the wallow. Only some fast acrobatics prevented me from ending up completely submerged. I came up spluttering, covered with slime. I stunk like I had never stunk before.

Old Maid Belle just glared at me as I rose up out of the hog wallow with the stinking mess dripping off my clothes, my hands, and even my face. I stuck my tongue out to wet my lips. It was on my lips and tasted horrible. I quickly drew my tongue back into my mouth. The hog had managed to dislodge the wire by now and stood under the shed warily watching me, that strange creature who had invaded its home.

"Miss Dawson, I don't think I'm going to be able to catch your hog."

"I don't think you are either, young man. It was sure a waste of time to have you come out." She ignored my condition.

"Let's wait and see if the hog doesn't get all right."

"If I have to get a vet back, I'll get Armer. You aren't going to charge me anything, are you?"

"You do owe for a trip, Miss Dawson," This was ludicrous. Here I was in the middle of a wallow in a stinking condition and arguing over whether a service fee was due or not.

I waded over to the fence and climbed out of the pen. "Miss Dawson, do you have anything I can clean up with?"

"There's some burlap sacks out in the barn. I'll talk to Armer about the charges." She turned her back on me and walked back towards her house.

"They just don't teach these youngsters anything in school anymore," I heard her muttering as she departed. As I entered the barn to try to find something with which to wipe the filth off, I heard the back door to her house slam. It was obvious that I had lost a client.

Silas Jackson Was a Big, Big Man

SILAS Jackson was a big, big man. He weighed over three hundred pounds but had the height to carry the weight. To go with his towering appearance, he had a booming voice. He dominated every conversation both physically and audibly. Si had worked as an engineer. He served as an officer in the U.S. Engineer Corps during World War I. Later he worked on construction projects in the United States. He told of working crews of men laying railroad track under the blazing summer Nevada sun. The secret of men working and surviving under those conditions, according to Si, was to wear long-john underwear and heavy long-sleeved shirts, drink plenty of water, and consume large quantities of salt. By doing so, the sweat-soaked clothes would keep a man cool on the hottest day and the water and salt would prevent heat stroke.

During the Depression Si returned to the family homestead to establish a registered Hereford operation. The Jackson ranch rapidly became known for the quality of its calves. They were especially in demand by 4-H members wishing to fatten calves for the county fair competitions.

Bert Douglas, the foreman, and his family lived on the ranch. Si was a widower and lived in town. Along with a booming voice, Si had an extraordinary command of swear words. Profanity was a part of nearly every sentence he uttered. Originally there had been a telephone at the ranch house but, because of Si's insistence on coloring the English language with the words and phrases he had picked up during his many years in the army and on construction projects, the telephone was disconnected. The telephone company explained to Si that the operators refused to service his calls because of his shocking language. Either eliminate the profanity from his telephone conversations or no telephone. Si was not about to be ordered around—so no telephone. This meant that the family living on the neighboring farm had to act as a go-between on telephone conversations between Si and his foreman. If the ranch had been two miles closer to town, Si's voice would have carried and the telephone would not have been necessary.

Over the years Si had developed a tremendous capacity for hard liquors. It was said he drove to Joplin, Missouri, for a case every two weeks. As far as I know, no county sheriff ever had the temerity to question Si's legal right to keep that quantity of whiskey in "dry" Kansas. Si would probably have torn the cell apart if they had ever taken him in—if they could have gotten him that far. He said he had his first drink as an eye-opener upon arising and it was reported he nipped all day long. Despite his awesome consumption, I never saw him under the influence. And, he survived beyond the average span of life. His liver had extraordinary regenerative powers.

My first close contact with Si's operation was as a result of being requested by Dr. Harry Cox, the district federal veterinarian, to be present at Si's ranch the next Friday. He was going to be reading the TB test on Si's herd at that time. It was injected on Tuesday because of tuberculosis found at slaughter in some 4-H stock that had been purchased from the herd.

Dr. Cox's father, Ed, had been a state veterinarian in the area. He and my father had worked together for years on various projects including one to determine if the "botting" of horses would reduce the incidence of swamp fever, scientifically known as infectious equine anemia. The state was paying indemnities on swamp fever cases at that time. It was suspected that the diagnosis was unreliable and that the state was paying for many animals that were sick or dying from other diseases. To test this hypothesis in relation to bot infection as a contributing factor, the state arranged through Dr. Ed for my father to be paid for botting horses in a designated area to see if it would reduce the incidence of swamp fever. The owners were required only to have the horses confined at the designated time and pay for the medicine. Bots were a stomach parasite and the program did yield positive results. Over the years the Coxes and the Porters became close friends and, when Harry and I returned to the area, this friendship was extended into the second generation. I later worked under Dr. Harry in Mexico on the foot-and-mouth disease eradication program.

Dr. Harry had visited with Si the previous week and gained consent to do the testing. A court order could have been secured to do the testing because bovine tuberculosis was under a state-federal eradication program. However, voluntary cooperation was desirable and practically always could be secured. Si had agreed to have the cattle confined and have the necessary manpower available to assist with the injections and with the reading of the test injections on the designated days.

One of the reasons Dr. Harry approached the Porters was to have a local veterinarian present just in case a significant amount of tuberculosis was found and he had to condemn and brand Si's cattle. When Dr. Harry had visited Si he had been impressed by Si's size, by his command of profanity, by his dislike of governmental controls, and by his consumption of liquor. Dr. Harry was apprehensive about what might happen if Si didn't approve of what could happen.

Si, on the other hand, didn't just dislike government officials. He hated them with a passion and had a special vocabulary of profane words to describe the "meddlers." While agreeing to cooperate with the testing, he had serious reservations about what might happen. He had confidence in my father, so he, like Dr. Harry, approached the Porters privately.

"Armer, that God damned federal veterinarian from Chanute is coming out to test my cattle next week," he said. My father and I said nothing about Dr. Harry having been by to see us. "Those S.O.B.s don't have anything better to do with their time than to bother us taxpayers who are trying to earn an honest living. During the last war they were trying to take ration points away from me because I butchered my own steer and stored the meat in my locker down at the slaughter house. Damn if I was going to give them the ration points. It was my meat, wasn't it? That secretary down at the board office, Mary Black, the one that's married to Tom Black's son, Bill; that stupid pen pusher tried to tell me that they wouldn't give me any ration points if I didn't agree to their withholding of points for my meat in my locker. Imagine her telling me what to do with my meat. I told her to take those points and ram them. Damn! This country has been going downhill ever since the Democrats got in back in Washington. Franklin wasn't the man his cousin, Teddy, was. By God, Washington ought to get off our backs so we could go to work. Those — — — ." He used some particularly strong words to describe the federal bureaucracy. My mother was in the next room and closed the intervening door so she wouldn't hear any more.

"Armer, I want you or Junior out at my ranch next Friday when that federal vet comes back to read the test. By God, I want him to know that I can have somebody watching over his shoulder."

My father agreed that one of us would be there. I got the assignment. The next Friday dawned bright and beautiful. A day so beautiful could hardly harbor any dire events. Besides, tuberculosis was nearly eradicated. Si's cattle were show quality. They couldn't have TB, so I relaxed and prepared for an uneventful day. I arrived at the ranch about 9:00 A.M. They told me it would take until about then to have the first groups of cattle corraled. Dr. Harry's car was parked by the chute, so I parked my car by the pasture gate, let myself through a couple of gates, and walked over to join him. Si wasn't to be seen.

Most of the cattle were rounded up. Dr. Harry was standing beside the head catch talking to Bert, the foreman, and to Sam Fink, who would man the head catch. The head catch was located on the end of a fifty-foot-long chute. The chute was narrow enough so adult cattle could not turn around. It was six feet high, constructed of solid hedge posts set upright in the ground six feet apart, to the inside of which were bolted two-by-four planks running horizontally the length of the chute and spaced four inches apart. Two men were leaning a large number of sections of heavy posts or two-inch pipe at intervals against the outside of the chute. The poles, as they were called, would be used in front of and behind animals in the chute to separate them. When the chute was filled with cattle, the two men working the chute would slip poles through the spacings separating the horizontal two by four in front of and in back of each upright post. This would separate each animal. If the animal was cantankerous and tried to climb over or crawl under the restraining pole, additional poles could be placed above or below the other poles to form an adequate barrier to restrain the animal. When they desired to move the animals forward, the poles would be removed and then reinserted as each animal was moved forward.

The chute led off from one of the four pens of the corral. The pens were connected to each other by gates so that cattle could be worked around to the pen that emptied into the chute. The pen from which the chute projected had a wing leading from one side of the entrance into the center of the pen. The opposite side of the entrance was continued by the corral fence. Thus the wing and one side of the pen were constructed in such a manner that they formed a funnel to assist in driving the cattle into the chute. The sides of the pens of the corral and of the projecting wing in the one pen were also six feet high and constructed of two-by-four boards horizontally spaced about eight inches apart.

The cattle were milling about in the pens and bawling incessantly. Many of the cows were separated from their calves in the turmoil and were frantically searching for their offspring. They didn't like being driven in from the pasture. They were apprehensive about what lay ahead. They had been through that chute three days before. They didn't like it, and they were letting everybody within hearing distance know of their displeasure.

"A little noisy here this morning," Dr. Harry shouted to me. We carried on much of our conversation by shouts because of the noise.

I nodded to the three men. "Didn't have any trouble getting them in?"

"You're damn right we did. They were spooky after Tuesday. The herds from the west pasture broke back twice before we got them through to the pasture here by the corral. Finally had Ralph and Bob drive some of the calves through to get the mothers to follow." Bert was speaking. "We kept the bulls up in the dry lot for the three days so we wouldn't have any trouble with them."

"Has Mr. Jackson showed up yet?" I inquired.

"No. He'll be along later," Bert promised.

"Bert, are you ready to go?" Dr. Harry was speaking.

"Sure. Might as well get started. It sure isn't going to get any quieter until we move some of these cattle back to pasture."

"O.K. Let's run the bulls. The thirteen of them are in the first pen."

"Polers ready?" Bert shouted to the two men along the chute.

"Polers ready," the men shouted back in unison.

Four men were sitting on top of the fence of the first pen. One of them was rolling a cigarette. He had the tobacco pouch held between his teeth while he manipulated the paper and tobacco with his two hands, rolling up the cigarette. This done, he held the newly rolled cigarette in one hand while he replaced the tobacco pouch in his shirt pocket with the other. Bert raised his hand above his head and moved it in a circle.

"Chutes ready! Roll 'em!" he shouted.

Three men jumped down into the pen with the snorting bulls. The man making the cigarette lingered on top to light it. The cigarette lit, he disappeared into the pen after his colleagues. A moment later he was scrambling back on top of the fence.

"Hey, Bill, you're not supposed to let those bulls scare you," Ralph's voice could be heard taunting him.

"I ain't scared. My feet are scared. My feet just won't listen to me."

"Get a club and get back in there. Tell your feet you got a club. We haven't got all day." A poler passed a stout club up to him and he disappeared back into the bull pen.

They got the bulls circling in the right direction and were able to head about half of them into the chute on the next try.

"Fire in the hold! Fire in the hold!"

Everybody could hear the lead bull snorting and his feet pounding on the packed ground as he raced down the chute heading for daylight. Seven other bulls were pressing behind him. The drivers were whooping to keep them moving. Each poler clutched a pole, ready to slide it in at the appropriate place.

"Ready, Sam. Here he comes."

Sam spit on his palms and rubbed them together. He grabbed for the rope that hung from the neck bar above. The bar could be pulled down on the upper side of the neck when the animal stuck his head through the V-shaped opening that formed the lower part of the head catch. This effectively restrained the animal's head while the necessary manipulations were being made.

"I never missed one yet, have I, Bert?"

The bull's head was through the head catch. He never slowed down. His front feet were off the ground. He was coming through. Sam brought the neck bar down on top of the bull's neck. His neck was forced down into the V. The bull came to a sudden halt and the whole front end of the chute vibrated. The other bulls piled in behind and were practically on top of each other before settling down and spreading back along the chute. The polers were busy poling the bulls apart so they could be worked individually. It all happened in less than a minute.

"Good chute you got there, Bert," Dr. Harry commented.

"You ought to say something about the good man Bert has catching those fireballs," Sam chimed in.

"By God, you do all right, Sam. I'd take you on my crew any day," Dr. Harry responded.

Dr. Harry was climbing up on the side of the chute to examine the right caudal fold on the confined bull. The caudal fold of skin runs down from the tail head to the perianal region on each side. He had injected tuberculin intradermally in that fold of skin three days before.

"Dr. Porter, come here and take a look."

I had never seen a tubercular reaction. The national testing program had reduced the number of tubercular cattle to the extent that many young veterinarians like myself starting out often had no experience with the disease. At one time tuberculosis in cattle posed a serious public health problem, thus the national disease eradication program. The program had succeeded to the extent that tuberculosis in man of bovine origin is seldom seen anymore. However, it had not succeeded in completely eradicating the disease, even though many of us young veterinarians had never seen it. Constant vigilance was and is necessary to prevent it from becoming a major problem again. Diligent efforts were and are being directed towards final eradication of the disease.

I had been conducting annual TB tests on local dairy herds and found nothing resembling a reaction. Wilson County was supposed to be clean. I expected to see nothing that day. It was too beautiful a day.

"Climb up here and feel this tail. You'll never see a better reaction." The entire right caudal fold of skin was swollen, hot, and red. "It's a beaut, isn't it?"

I nodded and tried to look intelligent as I palpated the fold of skin. "I never felt one before."

"Take a feel of those tails on the others poled off."

I walked back along the chute looking at or feeling the tails of the other seven bulls poled off. Three others had large visible swellings. Two more had palpable swellings. I was astounded.

Dr. Harry was getting a torch from his car. In a few minutes he had it fired up and was heating a branding iron marked with a T to a reddish glow. He pulled the bull's head around to the right with a nose lead and had Bert hold it while he applied the hot brand to the left jaw. The smell of burnt hair and hide filled the air. The bull opened his mouth, protruded his tongue, and loudly bellowed. The other bulls bellowed back in reply. This was going to be a noisy and a long day. Dr. Harry then put a reactor tag in the bull's ear. The reactor tag number and the bull's tattoo were recorded in his record book.

"He's got a lot of meat on his rear end, Doc. You sure he's got TB?" Sam was smiling as he addressed Dr. Harry.

"He may not be physically sick, but I wouldn't advise you to eat the meat," Dr. Harry replied.

"I don't think Si is going to like this," Sam added.

"I expect it will be a bad day for him. Did you glance at the tails of the cattle as they were being driven in?"

"Well, some did look a little large. This may be a two fifths day for Si."

"Did you ever see Mr. Jackson angry?" Dr. Harry asked the question.

"Shucks, the way he talks most of the time, I can't tell," Sam responded. "I have never seen him drunk either, but this may be his day."

"I sure wouldn't want to tangle with a man his size," Dr. Harry added.

"You may have to. Here he comes now." Bert had been watching down the road and spied Si's black Hudson coupe coming.

"You had better get your car started and leave it idling just in case you have to make a fast getaway." Sam was taunting Dr. Harry.

Dr. Harry smiled but didn't respond. One of the men crawled out of the pens and ran to open the gates for Si. In a few minutes his Hudson was parked besides Dr. Harry's car.

He opened the car door and cautiously eased himself out. He had to do it carefully because of his size. He was too tall for the car, especially with his Stetson hat on. He said he didn't necessarily prefer Hudsons but that Hudsons were the only modern car with enough head room for him. "They're building cars for midgets now."

Si dressed the part of a cattleman. He wore a suit coat, a string tie, and capped it off with a Stetson hat. He adjusted his hat after stepping out of the car and assumed his natural stature. He towered over everyone.

Si didn't say anything. He walked over and looked at the brand on the jaw of the animal and then looked at Dr. Harry. His silence was impressive, even with the cattle bawling. He remained silent and continued to stare. Dr. Harry saw that he was going to have to broach the subject. He fidgeted for a few minutes with some equipment, then stared up at Si. If he was going to die, he might as well do it bravely.

"Mr. Jackson, I hate to be the one to bring you bad news but this herd has tuberculosis and lots of it. This one has a large swelling under the tail and you can glance over the fence at the others. Many of them have swellings large enough to detect without feeling.

Si said nothing. After holding eye contact with Dr. Harry for a few minutes, he looked over at me. I looked back and smiled weakly. He turned and strode along the chute looking at the tails on the bulls. He then climbed the fence of one of the pens that held a milling group of cows and calves and looked down at them. He nodded over to some of the men in the adjoining pen.

"It looks like it's going to be a long day. Can your wife and kids handle the milking and chores at home this evening?"

"Sure they can, Mr. Jackson. The cows are about dry now, anyway."

"Mr. Jackson, I'll slip over to Ralph's at noon and call our wives. We're all on the same party line so it'll just take one ring."

"Just say we have a lot of cattle to work. Don't say anything about tuberculosis. It's premature yet."

"Sure, Mr. Jackson."

Si climbed down and walked back to the front of the chute. "Bert, does Sadie have enough food to feed this crew at noon? I can bring something back from town if she needs it."

"You brought plenty yesterday, Mr. Jackson. Bob's wife, Myrtle, came over to help with the cooking. There won't be any problem."

Si nodded to the rest of us and returned to his car. Ralph climbed over the fence and ran to open and close the gates as Si drove back to town.

Dr. Harry looked over at Sam with a questioning look.

"Just wait until he returns. He just went back to town to get another fifth. This is going to be a two fifths day for him."

"I guess he'd have a reason," Dr. Harry agreed. "I'm through with this bull for now, Bert. Ready to let it go?"

"Ready. We'll keep all the bulls together in the dry lot until Si tells me what to do with them. Let him go, Sam. We've got a long day ahead."

"Polers ready?" Sam shouted.

"Polers ready," they replied.

The neck bar was raised, releasing the bull's head. The bull had been pulling back trying to get loose. The sudden release caused it to stumble back until its rear end contacted the cross poles.

"Get that gate open! Here he comes!" Bert was urgently shouting to Sam.

Sam hurriedly pulled the bolt holding the head catch gate fast to the front end of the chute and swung the gate open. It swung free on the hinges supporting it on the opposite side of the front of the chute. While the gate was swinging open the bull started its forward charge. The gate had scarcely opened sufficiently to allow the unimpeded exit of the bull when it charged by snorting and swinging its head. Sam had ducked back for safety, and Bert swiftly swung the open gate back towards Sam.

"Fasten that gate fast, Sam. Those other bulls are climbing over each other trying to follow that first bull."

"Get high! Here he comes! He's looking for blood!" Bert was shouting a warning to Sam.

The released bull was stopped short by a fence at the other end of the lot. He turned and looked back at his tormentors. His jaw still hurt where it was branded. He was mad. He put his nostrils to the ground, snorted, and pawed the ground, warning those men back at the chute. When he looked up, the men were still there. He let out a bellow and charged. I started climbing. Sam had his back to the bull. He was slapping the restraining bolt for the chute gate back into its catch and didn't see the bull. When Bert gave the warning cry, Sam looked over his shoulder and started scrambling. The bull passed directly under Sam's feet. He dashed on along the outside of the chute shaking his head at the polers perched out of reach. Circling he headed back towards where Sam was roosting on top of the chute. This time the bull didn't stop. He slammed into the chute evidently planning to topple his tormentor. The chute vibrated but Sam grabbed an adjoining upright post and held on for dear life. The bull backed off a couple of steps so that he could better eye Sam while he snorted and pawed the ground.

"Ride'im, Sam!"

"Hell, you ride him. I've retired from bull riding."

The bull charged and slammed his head against the chute again.

"Want my spurs, Sam? They're offering one hundred dollars added money in the bull riding over at Elk City. Here's your chance to practice."

"You ride him. I'm a bull catcher, not a bull rider."

In the meantime, while the bull's attention was riveted on Sam, Bert climbed down and ran over and opened the gate into the adjoining pasture. He shouted back at the bull from the far side of the fence. By then the bull was losing interest in the man perched above. He looked toward the other man shouting at him and saw the open gate. After a final snort at Sam's boots, he whirled and raced through the open gate into the pasture. After the bull passed, Bert rejoined the group now climbing down from the fence.

"Let's get started. We've got a lot to work today yet," Bert ordered.

The polers released the next bull. It charged the opening in the head catch and was caught by Sam, his composure now recovered. It, too, was a reactor and was branded and tagged by Dr. Harry.

When released, it headed for the open gate and freedom. Eight of the thirteen bulls were reactors and were handled accordingly. After they were worked, the gate into the pasture was closed. Next, one of the pens of cows and calves was driven into the chute pen to be worked. The percentage of reactors in this group was comparable to that in the group of bulls.

Two hours later I saw Si's car coming back up the road.

"Here he comes."

"Dr. Cox, you'd better be ready to make a fast exit," Sam was chiding him again. "Si will be started on his second fifth by now."

Dr. Harry smiled back at him. "Mr. Jackson's bark is worse than his bite."

"Don't you believe it. Nobody has ever branded his cattle on the jaw before."

"Well, I guess my wife can collect on my government insurance policy if something happens. I may be worth more dead than alive."

"I'll give you two to one odds that she collects. How much do you want to take at those odds?" Sam asked.

"The government doesn't allow us to gamble on the job," Dr. Harry responded evasively.

Sam looked over at me. "Want some money at those odds? Dr. Cox to return to Chanute in a hearse?"

I negatively shook my head. "No thanks, Mr. Fink."

"Sam is my name. Nobody will know who you're speaking to if you say Mr. Fink."

By this time Si had driven up and joined us. Again he said nothing. His silence and physical stature dominated the scene. Dr. Harry had just finished branding a cow. The smell of burnt hair drifted up to Si's nose and he turned his head. Dr. Harry seized this slight advantage to initiate the conversation.

"About two-thirds are reactors, Mr. Jackson. We've run about seventy-five through so far and forty-eight were positive."

"I suppose you know what you injected into my cattle, Dr. Cox?" Si asked.

"Yes, sir." Dr. Harry took advantage of the opportunity to explain how tuberculin was produced.

"How many reactors did you ever see in one herd before?"

"Seven," Dr. Harry answered, "but this is good tuberculin." He didn't like the drift the conversation was taking.

Si walked over to me. "What does it look like to you, Dr. Porter?"

"Well, I slipped over to Smith's place and phoned my father. He stopped by and confirmed the swelling as tubercular reactions."

Satisfied since Dr. Armer had confirmed the reactions as tubercular, he walked back to his car, folded himself back inside and drove back towards town.

"Now he's really going to get plastered," Sam advised Dr. Harry. "You'd better finish and get out of here before he returns."

"Well, the federal and state governments will pay indemnities on these cattle."

"Si wants the cattle, not your money," Sam pointed out. "I'm advising you to be gone before he returns."

After finishing that pen of cows and calves, Bert ordered the men to stop for dinner. I excused myself and drove back to town.

Late that evening Dr. Harry stopped by. One hundred and sixty-three of 259 had shown reactions. It was the most reactors that Dr. Harry had ever heard of being found in one herd. Si had returned once more during the afternoon, and Dr. Harry stopped at his house before coming by my place. If he was drunk, Dr. Harry said he couldn't detect it.

"Furthermore, he offered to cooperate in whatever had to be done. If I had been in his shoes, I would probably have been drunk by that time. You should have taken some of the money that Sam was offering."

"What happens now?"

"There's nineteen cattle over in another pasture we can't get to until the week after next. After that the state appraiser comes down and he, the county commissioners, and Si will agree on a price. The federal pays one-third, the state pays one-third, and the owner stands one-third loss up to $75 on grade stock and up to $150 on registered stock. The cattle are always appraised at the top figure cited so the owner will lose the minimum possible. After that they are shipped to a federally inspected packinghouse for slaughter and postmortem examination."

We discussed where the disease had come from. Si had started the herd after the county had undergone the original countywide TB test and had been accredited. Dr. Harry said that Si had purchased part of his foundation stock from a herd out near Dodge City that was later found to be tubercular, but somebody had been lax in tracing dispersements from the herd. All sales should have been traced to the new owners and their herds tested. If that had been done with Si's herd, this catastrophe would probably have been avoided. One of the things that came out in the conversation was that Si's father's herd had extensive TB years before. Si thought the reason was because they were barned all winter. Consequently, Si insisted that the cattle in his herd be wintered outside.

In discussing the future, Dr. Harry stated that the herd had to be tested every sixty days and to pass two consecutive negative tests before it would be released from quarantine. Later, it would be tested annually for as long as the government felt necessary. Further, Dr. Harry explained it would be necessary to test every herd of cattle in the county immediately in order to retain accreditation. To do otherwise would mean that restrictions would be placed on the movement of cattle from the county. Accreditation required that the percentage of reactors must be less than 0.5% and that a certain percentage of the cattle be tested at specified intervals. In this case the number of reactors would require a test of all herds in the county. To do the necessary testing, every available government veterinarian in Kansas would be moved into the county. As they would still be short on help, I would be needed and would be paid on a service fee by the state of Kansas. Later, Dr. Harry excused himself and drove back to Chanute. I went to bed that evening still amazed at what I had witnessed that day.

Three weeks later Si stopped by my place with a rail ticket for me. Five carloads of his cattle were to be shipped to the Kansas City stockyard the next Monday night for slaughter on Tuesday. The railroad allowed one passenger ticket per carload of cattle. Nobody else was interested in going but Si wanted me to go.

The next Monday the reactor cattle were trucked into the railroad stockyards at Fredonia to be loaded. After the loading, I boarded the caboose and accompanied the switchmen on the nightlong ride into Kansas City. I was told after arrival that the cattle would be slaughtered by Armour after all the other cattle were slaughtered that day. There were four packing houses in Kansas City and the veterinarians from all four houses would be transferred into Armour at the close of their regular kill so the cattle could be processed as rapidly as possible. Accordingly, I took my suitcase and went out to my wife's aunt to find a bed for the night.

Late that afternoon I returned to Armour's packing house to observe the postmortem examination of the cattle. I should inform the reader that all tubercular reactors are not condemned to tankage. All organs and lymph glands are incised and examined for lesions by the inspectors. If no lesions are found, the carcass is passed for food. If localized lesions are found, the carcass is passed for food minus the localized areas of infection or passed for food after cooking. If extensive lesions are found, the carcass is condemned.

I expected to see a group of veterinarians when I arrived at the cattle floor; namely, the full force of federal meat inspectors stationed in Kansas City. I did not expect to see the additional veterinarians that also were there. Word had spread that 166 tubercular reactors were to be killed. All veterinarians in the area who had an interest in tuberculosis were present. The veterinarian who most attracted my attention was Dr. L. M. Roderick, my pathology professor from Kansas State College. Dr. Roderick always had a dour countenance; I had never seen him smile. That day he stationed himself on the walkway behind the veterinary inspectors. He had a washtub beside him. As the carcasses and organs came by and were examined, he salvaged organs with extensive lesions and dropped them in his washtub. That day he had a smile on his face that extended from ear to ear. Never before had he or any other Kansas State pathologist had the opportunity to collect such beautiful specimens and in such quantity. The pickle jars of organs in the pathology department would finally have a proper complement of specimens of tuberculosis. I can imagine him back at Kansas State that night processing the specimens, still with the big grin on his face. Every cloud has a silver lining. Pathologists must look for silver-lined clouds in order to get teaching materials.

Of the 166 reactors, 163 were from the one day and 3 from the test two weeks later; 7 showed no visible lesions, 107 showed lesions but were not condemned in total. Forty-nine showed lesions and were condemned in total, and 3 died before slaughter. Because of the persistence of tubercular reactors in the herd despite tests and slaughter of reactors, the herd was dispersed for slaughter fifteen months after the testing started.

This chapter would not be complete without relating what happened to Si Jackson and his dream. After the last of his herd was sent to slaughter, his apparent strong constitution began deteriorating and he died shortly thereafter. I never heard him complain about the federal veterinarian's activities, even though a laxity by some individual(s) had led to the overlooking of his herd as a possible harborer of tuberculosis until it had gained a strong and ineradicable foothold. He was a big man when I first knew him. He remained a big man in my eyes even in his last days. His is probably a perfect example of how a person with a dream and a purpose will live far longer than a person who does not have such objectives.

Wolf-in-the-tail

I honked as I drove by the house. Wes Smith had phoned the office earlier requesting that I stop by that morning to see a sick steer of his. He would be waiting at the house. I stopped at the barn and got out of the car. When I looked back towards the house, I saw Wes coming out the back door. Wes was an elderly, reddish-faced man of medium build. He had been farming and handling livestock years before I was born. Wes was a follower, not a leader—and he followed years behind. He was the last one in the area to purchase a tractor. He weaned calves and castrated and dehorned them by the signs of the moon. I should note that many other farmers—like many city people—also believed in the signs and wouldn't think of embarking on a serious undertaking without consulting the almanac. Wes, unlike his neighbors, still practiced many of the treatments for animals that had long since been relegated to the history books. To listen to Wes was to be exposed to the lore of my grandfather's day. I always picked up a few gems of historical knowledge when I called on Wes.

"Doc, the steer's tied up in the barn. I'll be there as soon as I fire up Ol' Betsy."

Wes remained on the back porch while he filled the bowl of his pipe with tobacco from a Prince Albert can carried in a pocket of his bib overalls. After tamping the tobacco down with his index finger, he shook some more tobacco on top and tamped again. Satisfied after careful inspection, he closed the lid on his Prince Albert can and returned it to the appropriate pocket. From another pocket he brought a stick match, which he proceeded to strike on the sole of his shoe. He held the burning match over the bowl of his pipe and took a few deep draws. Smoke rolled out of his mouth, the tobacco glowed, and a stream of smoke curled upwards out of the bowl. He grunted contentedly. Wes always followed this routine unless the wind was blowing too hard. Today, only a light breeze was blowing across the north 40, the pipe was drawing good; there was nothing to distract him from the task ahead. He headed for the barn to confront me, the vet with the book learning. The steer wasn't responding to lard and turpentine so he decided to invest some money in a college veterinarian. He meant to get his money's worth.

I had already entered the barn. It was sometimes wise to survey the situation before the owner arrived. The door opened onto a narrow walkway between a row of box stalls on one side and a row of stanchions on the other. The steer was tied loose in a box stall. On the opposite side of the walkway, a cow was confined with her head in a stanchion. Wes usually had a second or even a third animal confined for me to look at as long as I was coming out. It was cheaper that way.

"Didn't think it was worth a special trip, Doc, but Spot hasn't been doing well," he would say. "She has 'wolf-in-the-tail' just like Blacky had a couple of years ago. I tried some of Dr. Smith's Elixir on her. I've been using that elixir on 'wolf-in-the-tail' for years just like my pappy and grandpappy before me but Spot just isn't improving. Why don't you look at her as long as you are here?"

I had my back to Spot and was making a cursory survey of the steer from the walkway. Wes had just entered the doorway. At this moment, the cow humped up, raised her tail, and proceeded to urinate on my back. I was looking at the steer and wasn't prepared to take evasive action.

"Har! Har! Doc, she remembers that needle you jabbed her with the last time you were here."

I didn't think it was funny. I was soaked but I wasn't going to show my irritation in front of Wes. After all, I had committed a cardinal sin by turning my back on the cow's rear feet. She could have kicked me. "Well, the next time I'll use my blunt needle," I countered.

"Better not let her hear you say that or she'll do both jobs on you next time," Wes chuckled.

Wes was feeling good. His pipe was drawing good. The vet had gotten his comeuppance. Wes was looking forward to discussing the diagnosis of the steer's ailment.

I turned my attention to the steer. After taking the temperature rectally (animals don't cooperate with the taking of oral temperatures), listening to the heart and lungs with a stethoscope, feeling over the left flank for movement of the rumen, and looking as professionally dignified as possible in a cow barn, I pronounced that the steer had impaction. That meant that the rumen was packed with too much dry roughage and the steer needed a laxative.

"That's what I told the wife. He's got dry murain. Think we ought to drench him with a dose of salts?"

"I've got something better. Get me a bucket of water."

"Sure you don't want to use the salts? I've got some up at the house."

"Wes, I think you've been using salts and it hasn't worked. We'll use my medicine this time. Get me a bucket of water."

Wes left muttering under his breath that the steer needed salts. When he returned with the bucket of water, I dissolved some medicine that Wes couldn't recognize in it. I then inserted a mouth gag into the steer's mouth and passed one end of a stomach tube through the opening in the gag, down the esophagus, and into the rumen. After pumping the medicine through the stomach tube into the rumen, I withdrew the tube and removed the mouth gag. I then kneaded the flank area over the rumen for several minutes with as serious a countenance as possible. Wes would be expecting the full show or he would be complaining about the bill. I planned to head off his complaints on that score.

Next I looked at Spot. Wes knew she had "wolf-in-the-tail." Her back was humped up and she grunted when she walked. He knew those signs always went with "wolf-in-the-tail."

"How long has she been sick?"

"Oh, three or four weeks."

"See that humped back and swollen brisket?"

"Sure that goes with 'wolf-in-the-tail.' With 'hollow horn' they hold their head extended and their back isn't arched."

" 'Wolf-in-the-tail,' hell, she's got hardware. Here, I'll listen to her heart."

I bent over and listened with a stethoscope. A splashing sound could be clearly heard coming from the pericardial sac. There was no doubt. The cow had swallowed a piece of wire; it had worked forward through the wall of the recticulum, the second stomach, into the pericardial area. An infection had resulted and the purulent fluids were sloshing around with each beat of the heart. The cow was going to die.

"Wes, Spot isn't going to make it."

"Doc, you sure you shouldn't try some of that new drug—what do they call it—penicillin, isn't it? I hear it cures some real bad cases."

"It won't cure this case. Spot is going to die."

"Not on me, she won't. I'll haul her into Butch Kelsey's this afternoon for butchering."

"If you do, Armer will condemn her. Spot isn't fit for food."

"He wouldn't do that, would he? Hell, she's still go a lot of meat on her bones."

"If you want to eat her, that's your business, I guess. But you wouldn't want Sam Brown down the road to haul a cow in this condition into Dutch's and you end up buying the meat at the market, would you?"

"Doc, I can't afford to have this cow die on me. She's worth $150."

"Not now, she isn't."

"I suppose you want to be paid for the trip out here too. How am I going to do that if you won't let me sell Spot?"

"That's your problem, not mine. I do expect to be paid. The bill will be ten dollars."

After some grumbling about the unfairness of everything, Wes got out his checkbook and wrote me a check. I pocketed the check and drove back to town. It was typical of the experiences I had when I visited Wes's farm. Someday I should write a book about the ancient diseases and treatments propounded by Wes Smith so they wouldn't be lost to posterity.

That evening, as I was eating supper, the telephone rang. (Kansans eat supper not dinner in the evening; dinner is eaten at noon.) Marian answered the telephone. It was Wes wanting to know if Doc was home. Marian called me to the telephone. She was used to the meals being interrupted. In fact, she would have thought it unusual if the telephone hadn't rung while I was eating.

"Doc, remember that steer you doctored this morning?"

"Sure," I replied. I presumed the steer wasn't any better. I never received calls when the animals were doing all right. "How's the steer doing?" I prepared to listen to a long list of symptoms or a discussion of the relative value of salts compared to the medicine I had given.

"O.K., so far. It's too early to tell. That's not the reason I called." He paused for emphasis before continuing. "I took my wife to the doctor's this afternoon."

"Oh, I'm sorry. Is she getting along all right?"

"Yeah, I guess so, but I found out something else."

"What's that?" I knew he was baiting me. My curiosity was aroused, though, so I bit.

"Well, Dr. Miller didn't charge me as much as you did."

"Oh." I began to get an inkling as to where the conversation was leading.

"That's right and if you think for one minute that I think more of my steer that I do of my wife, you've got another think coming." With that, he hung up before I could collect my wits to reply that I would have charged less if he had trucked the steer to my office—or that his wife didn't urinate on Dr. Miller—or that . . . I finished my supper in a foul mood.

Bugle Trees a Coon

MARIAN, this is Maud."

"Hello, Aunt Maud."

"Al told me to call and to tell you and Junior to come out tonight and go hunting with him. The weather is cold enough now so the dogs should trail good."

"I'd like to if I can keep up. I may not be up to all the running up and down hills they talk about."

"Don't let them fool you. I've been out with them. They just find a good spot and let the dogs loose. Most of the time they're sitting around a fire on top of a hill swapping stories and listening to the dogs trail. I think they get most of their enjoyment out of listening to the dogs baying."

"Well, O.K. What time will Uncle Al start out?"

"Why don't you and Junior come out for supper? That way you can get started before it gets too late. Al used to stay out as long as the dogs would last, but he's slowing down in his old age. He needs to get in bed by midnight if he's going to milk the cows before he starts work the next day. I can milk the cows but arthritis in my hands is slowing me down. I'd just as soon Al do it. You plan to sleep here tonight. It'll be too late to drive back to town."

"Well, if Jim gets in off the calls early enough, we'll come on out. Otherwise, I'll give you a ring. I don't think I can help very much with the milking though. When I tried last time we were there I could hardly get a squirt. I just don't have any grip."

"That's all right. It takes practice to milk. Al can do it. He's got sixty more years practice than you. We'll look for you tonight. Al is real anxious to start hunting again this winter. Say, Marian, if the line is busy when you call, just tell Josie, the operator, to break in. Some of the people on this party line can talk for hours if they aren't interrupted."

Marian hung up the receiver. She was new to country life. Uncle Al had told her the previous summer when he first met her that he would take her coon hunting this winter. His stories about the nights when they followed the baying of the hounds as they trailed the raccoons had intrigued her. She told him to call her when the hunting season started.

I did get caught up on the farm calls by late afternoon so turned the telephone answering over to Armer, Sr., and we drove out to Maud and Al's farm. Marian asked Armer if he wanted to go but Armer shook his head. "The arthritis in my hip is acting up. I don't think I'll try it tonight. Just don't fall in the river when you're crossing on some of those fallen trees. If you do, you'll get all wet and clothes just don't dry standing around a bonfire."

Marian promised that she would watch her step.

When we arrived at the farm, Marian found Maud in her kitchen. Though slightly built, Maud was wiry from years of farm activities. She was hurrying around getting the table set and frying some meat and potatoes in a skillet on top of the wood stove. "Got to put something inside you that will give you some energy. You can get cold and hungry out there tonight."

"I expect my feet are going to cause me more trouble than anything else. I did bring plenty of clothes and have some overshoes I can slip on."

"Marian, they're kidding you. There's more talking than walking. I do think you'd better take my boots though. They'll give you more protection than the overshoes in fording those creeks."

"O.K., if they'll fit. Let me help you set the table. Where are the plates and silver?"

"We'll just use the everyday plates from the kitchen cupboard over there if it's all right with you. You aren't company anymore. The silver is in the drawer underneath. How do you and Junior like your meat?"

"Well done. Jim has taken too much parasitology in school to enjoy the thought of eating raw meat."

"That's the same way Al likes it. In his case, he doesn't know anything about parasites but his dentures just can't handle raw meat. Slice some of that bread in the bread box and put it on the table. That's real bread, not store stuff. I baked it last Saturday."

"I'm going to have to get a starter from you one of these days and try my hand at baking bread. My father learned how to do it but I've never tried it yet."

"Anytime. I've had that starter going for several months now. It works real well."

Just then Al came in from the back porch. He was a large heavy-set man with a receding forehead like all of the Porters. We had heard the separator humming out there so I knew he was busy turning the crank that ran the separator. The separator was used to separate the cream from the milk, hence the name, separator. The method might seem primitive to us now but it was considered very advanced in those days. The alternative was to let the milk stand and the cream rise to the top naturally.

"Marian, ready to go catch that coon?"

"Yes, if you think I can keep up."

"Ol' Blue will do the running. You won't have to do much walking until he and Bugle get that coon treed."

"How do you know he's treed the coon?"

"By listening to his bay. There's nothing like Ol' Blue's bugle when he has a coon treed. It's one of the most beautiful sounds you'll ever hear."

"I guess our dog Mitzie will never be a coon dog. All she does is yip. I don't think she'd last very long on a trail."

"I don't know about her running but a coon would kill her in no time. If you want a coon dog, I'll look around for one you can buy at a reasonable price."

"No, thanks. I'll stick with Mitzie. If I decide to become a coon hunter after tonight, I'll talk to you then about getting a hound dog."

"We'll make you a coon hunter. You just wait."

We were now seated at the table, stowing away huge chunks of meat and potatoes between bites of bread spread with home-churned butter and washing it all down with swallows of hot coffee. When we had finished, Maud offered us some canned pears she had canned last fall.

"No, thanks," Marian replied. "If I eat any more I'll never be able to get out of this chair, let alone go hunting with the men."

"I invited Steve Parker, my neighbor over west, to go along," Uncle Al said. "He hunted with me last winter and has a good coon dog. His dog, Killer, is a natural coon fighter. Coons can bluff out lots of hounds but Ol' Killer will tackle them head on. She's got a few slits in her ears to show for it but she's never let a coon get away yet. The trouble with her ears is that they hang down too far. They are just too floppy for her to keep out of the way." Smiling a little at the contemplation of the future events of the evening, he walked over to the telephone hung on the wall and dialed three short rings.

"That you, Steve? Didn't know for sure. Sometimes Bob Story

picks up the receiver and I can't tell your voices apart. Oh hello, May . . . you say Bob's sick today. Sure sorry to hear it. What's his trouble this time? Are his gall stones acting up again? . . . You say it's his kidneys this time. That's what I had last summer. Makes you want to crawl up the wall, it does. Say, let me get through my conversation with Steve and I'll put Maud on the line to talk to you. Say, Steve, bring Killer and come on over. We're ready to go, over here. Who's that? . . . John . . . you say the George brothers caught three coons over on Jordan's north 40 last night. You think it might be a good spot to go to tonight . . . Maybe so, and then maybe they've scared all the other coons out of there . . . Well, thanks for the information anyway . . . I've got to go get my dogs leashed. I'll put Maud on to talk to May . . . So long." He handed the receiver over to Maud. "May wants to talk to you."

"May, I'll call you back later. I've got to get Junior's wife, Marian, bundled up and booted so that she can go with the men tonight. . . . Me, no, I quit going with Al. I'll call you back later."

Al was going out the back door to locate and chain his two hound dogs, Ol' Blue and Bugle. He attached a chain to the snap on their collars when he called them to eat the table scraps from supper. In the meantime Marian was being fitted with a pair of heavy socks and Maud's rubber work boots. I had my own rubber boots I used in my veterinary practice to wade through the muddy lots of my clients. A few minute later we heard the sound of the pickup's motor and then saw its lights as it approached on the road from the west. Ol' Blue picked up her head and started sniffing the air. Bugle let out a long, low, penetrating bay from her throat. Tails began to wag rapidly and the dogs started frantically jumping up and down at the end of their chain leashes. They sensed they were going hunting, and they were doing their utmost to assure Al they were eager and willing to go. It had been along time since the previous winter's hunting season. The truck approaching from the west pulled off the road and into the farmyard. It came to a halt in front of us and the dogs. Killer, chained in the bed of the pickup, was jumping up and down and bellowing his joy with short sharp yelps on seeing the other two dogs. They responded in a similar manner.

Steve opened the truck door and climbed down. By the dim ceiling light of the truck cab, we were able to see him. He wore a cap with ear muffs loosely hanging down from the cap. A heavy sheepskin coat, heavy work trousers, and knee-top rubber boots completed his garb. He was a slim, gaunt-looking man with a face reddened by years of outdoor living. Out of his mouth protruded a pipe. The smoke curling up out of the pipe's bowl gave off a pleasant aroma in the cool night air.

"Steve, you've met Junior before. This is Marian, his wife. She's never been coon hunting." Al was making the introductions. "I invited them out to initiate her."

"Glad to meet you, ma'am." Steve pulled off the glove from his right hand and stuck his hand out towards Marian. Like all farmers, the hand was well calloused from years of manual labor. "So you're Junior's wife. He knows how to pick them, doesn't he now?"

"I told you he did," Al was now speaking. "It's supposed to get down around fifteen or twenty degrees tonight. That ought to be a good temperature for the dogs to work."

"The temperature won't bother any. Some of the creeks may be frozen over so we can walk across on the ice now."

"I wouldn't trust the ice yet. Remember last year when you fell through on Big Sandy?"

"Well, it had thawed a little that day. I don't plan to take any chances tonight; it's too hard to get clothes dried out."

By that time all the dogs were chained in the pickup bed. The four of us climbed up into the cab. Al had assured us it wasn't far so Marian was sitting on my lap.

Al mentioned that the George brothers caught three coons over on the Jordon's north 40 last night, according to John Mercer. Steve agreed with Al that the coons were probably staying out of that area for now. Al suggested that they try the hills over on the other side of Baker's Ford on the south fork of the Little Sandy. Steve allowed as to how they had had a good night over there last January so maybe it would be a good place to loose the hounds.

About fifteen minutes later we drove slowly through the water at Baker's Ford. We then followed a dirt road up through the hills overlooking the creek until we came to a six-strand, barbed-wire gate on the left side of the road near the top of a hill. I climbed out and opened the gate. After Steve had driven through, I closed the gate and climbed back into the cab with Marian again on my lap. The crest of the hill was covered with "black jack" oak trees. Steve drove the car along a dirt trail that skirted the tree-covered summit of the hill until he was on the south side of the hill.

"Let's loose the dogs here. This is the south side so these trees ought to give us some shelter from the north wind if it starts blowing." Steve had parked the pickup and he and Al climbed down and went around to the rear of the vehicle so that they could release the dogs. The dogs were on their feet, prancing and baying for all their worth. They knew their job and were eager to get started. When released they accepted a quick pat on the head and a few words of encouragement from their masters, then they were gone. Occasionally we could hear a quick bark but mainly nothing. The night was still and cold. We gathered up some fallen limbs by the aid of a flashlight and got a fire started by which we could keep our hands warm. Steve struck a match to relight his pipe. "Never smoked, did you, Al?" Steve asked.

"Yes I did. I got a cancer on my lip and had to have it cut out at Bell Memorial Hospital in Kansas City. Quit after that."

"I should quit but if I wasn't smoking I'd be chewing. Al, it sure is good to get out with the hounds again, ain't it?"

"It is, but I'll have to confess you about had me hunted out last winter. We went damned near every night that it wasn't storming and there weren't very many nights it stormed."

"Al, I thought you were the one who was eager to go. You called over every night."

"I guess I did but I'd tell Maud some nights before I called that I just about hoped you'd say you were too tired to go."

"That may be so but you've got at least twenty years on me and you were still out-hiking me on the way back to the pickup when we came in."

"That's right. I think hunting relaxes me. Actually I feel ten years younger every evening after listening to those hounds bugle. It's the the sweetest music this side of those angels' harps at the Pearly Gates."

Marian interrupted, "This is sure a funny way to go hunting. Do the dogs chase the coons back here to you?"

"No," Al chuckled. "We just wait until they tree a coon and then go to them."

"I still don't understand. How can you tell when they've treed a coon. I hear the dogs barking once in awhile but one bark sounds the same as the other."

"I can see you don't know hound dog talk yet. Just wait and listen. They are just scouting now. When they get a hot trail, they'll start baying in earnest. It's really beautiful to just listen to them chase the coon down. Those coons are smart though. They'll give the hounds the slip sometimes. You can tell by the hounds' uncertain barks that they're just trying to pick up a trail now. If we were following them we would be all tuckered out before the night was half over. There'll be time enough to catch up with them after they tree a coon. You'll know they've got a coon up a tree by their bugling."

"Yes, but what if they keep going in one direction and run out of hearing range?"

"Well, that does happen, but not often," Al was laughing. "If that does happen, why we just get back in the truck and head out that way until we hear them again."

"You mean to say you never lost a dog?"

"No, not really," Steve was speaking. "The few times we have lost them they were always home for breakfast the next morning."

"Well, there was that time that our hounds got mixed up with the hounds of the Roberts' boys one night. They ended up over at Jim Roberts' place over in Verdigris township and we had to go get them the next day. Remember?"

"Well, they still weren't lost. Remember Ken Roberts offered me three hundred dollars for Killer when I came for him. I suspect he killed the three coons they were bragging about bagging that night."

Marian interrupted again. "I haven't heard anything from the hounds for awhile. Are you sure they're still out there hunting?"

"They're there," Al answered. Just then one of the hounds started giving some yips. The second answered, and then the third. "That's Ol' Blue leading the way. She's got a whiff of a fresh coon trail. Just listen now."

No sooner had he finished speaking than we heard the yipping chorus of all three dogs as they seemed to be heading out in a westerly direction from where we were sitting. A few minutes later the chorus changed to a scattered yipping again. "They've lost the trail. The coon probably crossed over to the other side of Little Sandy and the dogs will have to pick up the trail on the other side."

The yipping of one hound did start in earnest later. The other two soon joined in the music and they seemed to be approaching again. "The coon did cross the creek. The hounds are trailing him back this way on the other side now."

"Steve, have you got your flashlight and .22 ready? We may be moving out in a few minutes." Al was speaking.

"I'm ready but don't get too anxious. They haven't treed him yet."

As if in answer to Steve's cautionary remarks, the steadying baying died away to interrupted yips. "Suppose they've got a skunk rather than a coon."

"They've got a coon. Ol' Blue won't trail skunks and she's the lead dog. I do remember though, when Junior was a kid, that Armer brought Junior, Margaret, and Laurine out one night and they and my kids went along with me and Armer hunting one night. I think little Ed Porter (they called him little Ed to distinguish him from big Ed, his cousin) came over and the Clark boys came up and we all went out. There must have been fifteen or twenty of us in the party and we were hoofing after the dogs down on Snake Creek. That was in my younger days when I was still a hiker. That was a civet cat night I'll always remember."

"A civet cat night. This is a story you haven't told me before," Steve said.

"It's a night I'd like to forget. Well, we got some time to wait before they get the coon treed from the sound of their barking. I might as well tell you about it. You remember that night, Junior?"

I hadn't spoken much for the last hour but the question did bring back some memories of a night almost forgotten. "Yes, I do remember. We had to hike back a couple of the miles to the house and you brought up the rear carrying that skunk."

"It was a civet cat, not a skunk. Civet cats stink worse. Well, Armer and Ed said since my dog had run it down, it was my responsibility to carry it in. They said they sure weren't going to let me lead the way with the civet cat. I was ordered to the rear—way back to the rear—so the odor couldn't be smelled by the others."

"Why did you carry it in?" Marian asked. "I would have wanted to get away from the smell as fast as possible."

"Furs were worth something in those days. Couldn't afford to throw it away. I remember when we used to cash in several hundred dollars worth of furs at the end of the hunting season. Cecil used to have a trap line he'd run. Made enough to buy his school clothes and then some—but not anymore. It's hardly worth while skinning these coons out. If it wasn't for the sport, I sure wouldn't do it now."

"If I had been Maud, I wouldn't have let you back in the house," Marian said.

"Well, she just about didn't," Al replied. "I had to undress outside in the cold and she made me chain the dog, Spot, out in the barn for the next week. Spot was always getting into trouble like that. He seemed to have a weakness for skunks."

"I think I'd have gotten rid of Spot," interjected Steve.

"Well I probably would have but he did get lost one night and never came back. I sure didn't look very hard for him."

"It saved you having to pay somebody to take him, huh?" chuckled Steve.

"Maybe so. The worst thing about those skunk dogs is that they'll teach the other dogs that bad habit. You just can't break them of chasing skunks once they get it in their blood."

"Oh, I don't know. I once had a dog, Sam. Now he was a skunk dog if there ever was one. My wife and I just about split up over that dog. She told me it was me or Sam. Hell, Sam was a good dog if I could just get him over chasing skunks. You know what I did to break him of that habit?"

"No, I sure don't," Al replied. "I didn't think they could be broke."

"I didn't either until then but it was me or Sam and Sam had a lot of potential."

"Well, what did you do?"

Steve laughed. "Well, I figured the only way to break him was to give him too much of what he thought was a good thing."

"How did you do that?" Al inquired.

"I shot one of those skunks he holed up and then just tied it to him in such a way he couldn't get it off. After about two weeks I cut it off, and he never wanted to look at a skunk after that."

"Your wife took you back, then?" Marian asked.

"Well, for twenty-five years she has." Steve continued. "I'm on my good behavior not to get another skunk dog."

Just then one of the hounds started giving out with a steady stream of yips. He sounded like he was on the other side of the next hill, maybe a half-mile away. For the next few minutes the yipping all came from the same area. Then, as if the dog had a hot trail again, the yipping started getting dimmer as the dog apparently followed a trail leading away from us. The other dogs soon joined in as they also picked up the trail and accompanied the other dog.

"That's Ol' Blue leading," Al was saying. "She's got a real nose on her. She may not be much of a scrapper after they get the coon treed, but she's sure responsible for getting a lot of coons treed."

The baying of the dogs indicated that the trail circled around a hill half to three-quarters of a mile away and was now headed back towards us.

"We've been here about an hour now," Marian said. "How long does it take them to tree a raccoon?"

"That's coon, not raccoon," answered Steve. "You never heard of raccoon hunters or raccoon hound dogs, now did you?"

"O.K. I'll learn. How long does it take for the dogs to tree a coon, then?"

"Well, I guess there have been nights when they never did tree a coon," Al replied. "As long as one has a fire to keep warm by, though, it hardly matters. The music is the thing. Now, I'd far rather listen to that hound dog music than I would to listen to that philharmonic music on the radio. Three or four hound dogs can make some real harmony."

The trail yipping stopped moving. The three dogs seemed to be barking as loud as they could in an area possibly a half-mile directly south of us. "On a clear night like this the sound really carries well. They've got that coon treed over in the hollow just south of the bend in the Little Sandy. There's a little grove of trees there, if I remember right," Al explained.

"You're right," Steve added. "The problem is how are we going to cross the creek? I believe there are some fallen trees down near the bend that we can climb across on. If we can't do that, we'll have to go back across the ford on the road and walk in from there."

"Let's try the tree crossing," Al said. "It will save a lot of time if we can do it. It might be an extra half-mile in from the road."

"O.K. I'm game if you are. Ready to go, Marian and Junior? This is what it is all about."

We ventured as to how we were, so Steve and Al stomped out the fire with their feet, threw some loose dirt on it, and we started down the hill. The fallen trees were located about where Steve had said they would be. After scouting the lay of the trees with flashlights, we decided we could climb across without too much difficulty. Even Marian thought she could make it. Steve climbed and walked across first, pipe clenched between his teeth, stepping gingerly from one limb to another while holding on to other limbs and climbing across other obstructing limbs where necessary. Marian, with Al's assistance, crossed next, aided by the light of flashlights directed by Steve and myself. It was left for me to join the others on the other side.

"Watch your footsteps as you're climbing over that limb out in the center. The limbs you're walking on are covered with ice. We don't want the last man to fall in." Steve was giving me some last minute advice as I pushed my flashlight back under my belt and started across.

I made it to the overhanging limb in the center without difficulty. I grasped an overhead branch and climbed over the obstructing limb. As my feet came down on the foot log on the other side, the log rotated and I found myself sliding into the icy water. I managed to catch myself but not until after my boots were filled with water and my pants and underclothes soaked. "Damn!" That was the only word that I could think of to express my feelings.

I climbed and splashed across to the other side where Steve and Al gave me helping hands to climb back out on the bank. "Now look who got wet," Marian scolded. "You were the one warning me to watch my step and now look."

"But the log rolled."

"I crossed on the same log and it didn't roll on me."

"You all right Junior, other than being wet?" Al was inquiring about my well-being.

"Sure, I'm all right except for having my feelings hurt."

"We'd better get the coon and get you back to the house. You aren't going to get dry out here."

While these events had been occurring, we could hear the frantic barking and baying of the hounds. They did have something treed. When we arrived at the scene, we found the hounds encircling a large cottonwood tree, barking at the top of their voices, and periodically standing on their hind legs with their feet frantically clawing the tree trunk above them as they sought a foothold to climb the trunk after the treed animal. A beam from the flashlight revealed a raccoon's head peering down from the first fork of the tree branches some thirty feet above us.

"What do we do now, Al?" Steve asked, "I'd sure like to see Killer tackle that coon but I don't know how we'll get him down alive. Besides, Junior is all wet and need to get him home to dry out before he catches his death of pneumonia."

"I think you'd better shoot the coon. We'll have other nights for coon fights," Al answered. "We'd better get Junior home or Marian won't ever go hunting with me again."

A well-placed shot between the eyes brought a dead raccoon falling at our feet. Al and Steve beat the dogs off with kicks and retrieved the carcass. After a few yips and loud barks the dogs became resigned to the fact that the raccoon was dead and quieted down.

Steve volunteered to go back and get the pickup and meet the rest of us when we walked out to the road. Some forty-five minutes later we met again on the main road. The hounds had followed us back. Al and Steve chained them in the truck bed, we climbed into the cab—me with my damp clothes and Marian on my lap—and returned to Al's home. After releasing the hounds and saying goodbye to Steve, Marian and I entered the house. Al took the raccoon out to hang in the barn.

Maud, clad in nightgown and robe, entered the front room where we were. "Well, how are the mighty hunters tonight?"

"Jim is all wet. Fell through up on Little Sandy."

"I see he is. I thought you were home a little early. Let me throw a couple of logs on the fire. Junior can change into some dry clothes of Al's and get warmed by the fire before you go to bed."

"Maud, can I fix some coffee? I think I need something to warm my insides and expect Jim does too."

"Sure, just dip some water out of the bucket by the wash stand. The coffee is in the cupboard over near the window. Here, Junior, slip into the other room and change into these clothes for now. I think they'll fit. You and Al are about the same size."

Just then Al entered the room. "I caught my first coon of the season, I did. Hung it up from the rafters in the barn. Guess it will wait until tomorrow for skinning. It sure isn't going any place now."

"I don't see why you bother to skin them. They don't hardly bring three dollars a fur now. Used to, you could get seven or eight dollars each," Maud said.

"I know, but my daddy taught me never to throw anything away. I guess I'll keep skinning them even if they don't give over fifty cents apiece for the skins."

"How come you let Junior get wet?"

"Now, Maud, I didn't have anything to do with it. You had better get him into some dry clothes though."

I reappeared from the next room. Later as we sat around the table nibbling on some chicken legs left over from a previous meal and swallowing some scalding coffee, Al and Marian were recapitulating the events of the evening.

"Uncle Al," Marian asked, "do you ever eat coon?"

"I sure do. We'll have some the next time you come out. It's possum I can't handle. Too greasy. Possum is southern food, but coon is good Kansas food."

Maud chimed in. "I think possum would be all right if you knew how to cook it. I've been told that you bake it with sweet potatoes. The potatoes soak up the grease."

"I don't think I want to try it," Marian said. "I might take Uncle Al up on his offer to eat raccoon, though."

"Marian, we don't have raccoons out here. Those are coons."

"I forgot, Uncle Al. I meant coons."

Sometime later as we were nestling down in bed in one of the upstairs bedrooms with a feather mattress and comforter, Marian said to me, "Maud gave me a chamber pot that is at the foot of the bed. I don't fancy traipsing out to the outhouse tonight. Besides, Maud says her grandchild, Betty, saw a copperhead snake in there last week. I'm not about to get bit by a snake in an outhouse."

I grunted, "They won't bite if you leave them alone!"

"They'd bite me. I sure don't want to be going outdoors tonight with a flashlight. I'd wake up Uncle Al's dogs."

"I think they're probably about asleep just like me," I yawned.

"Do you suppose there are scorpions in the outhouse, too? They're poisonous, too."

I didn't answer.

"Jim, how do I turn off this coal oil lamp? Aunt Maud said something about turning down the wick and then blowing it out. Jim, will you do it? I've never used these lamps before."

I didn't move. I was sound asleep.

Blood Transfusions and Blood Lines

SUMMERTIME was generally a slow time for a rural veterinarian. The stockmen did their routine veterinary work during the winter when it would not interfere with farming activities. Further, they needed surgery such as dehorning and knife castration done in the winter so that the wounds would be healed before fly season with the accompanying maggot or screwworm infection. Since then a governmental screwworm sterilization program has eradicated the pest.

However, epidemics did occur in the summer and when these occurred, there would be no rest for days. When I was a boy, horses were still the primary power source for the farmer. Sleeping sickness outbreaks in horses followed the seasonal increase in mosquitos. My father would drive all day making calls to treat the sick horses. When night came, my mother took over behind the wheel of the car and chauffeured my father until he finished the day's work. There were few miracle drugs in those days. However, the horses were worth a lot of money so everything possible was done to save their lives. Another problem that affected horses, this of a noninfectious nature, was heat stroke. Temperatures in excess of 100°F frequently caused this condition in horses being used in harvesting or plowing activities. Ice was a miracle drug in treating that condition if used promptly. My father would drive by the local ice plant and buy ice in 100 pound blocks to haul with him as he sped to the relief of the horses prostrated from overheat. Speeding consisted of possibly making forty-five miles per hour in a Model A Ford on the gravel or rutted dirt roads that existed; this was bone rattling speed. By the time I became a veterinarian the tractor had replaced the horse, causing a great decrease in the number of horses and an elimination of their use as draft animals. I haven't seen a heat stroke case in years and the development of sleeping sickness vaccine eliminated sleeping sickness epidemics.

Cattle and hogs also suffered from epidemics of infectious diseases. Yellow fever (anaplasmosis) often caused serious outbreaks in cattle in the late summer and fall. It was a parasitic disease that caused destruction of the red blood cells. This resulted in anemia and, in adult cattle, often death. Presumably the younger cattle had a higher potentiation for the production of red blood cells and thus didn't suffer symptomatically as did the adult cattle. The disease was transmitted mechanically by vectors carrying infected red blood cells from a carrier to a susceptible animal. Man might act as a vector if he didn't disinfect his instruments between dehorning or castrating operations. Insects, particularly horseflies (tabanids), were the natural vector.

When I started practicing, there was no way to treat the cattle except symptomatically although arsenic products were thought to have therapeutic value. During an outbreak the veterinarians would be busy until approximately thirty days after the first insect-killing frost, attempting to do what was possible to treat the sick cattle.

Theoretically, blood should have been an excellent supportive treatment since yellow fever caused illness because of the destruction of the red blood cells. Therefore, being a young and eager practitioner, I followed the lead of many of my colleagues and gave blood transfusions. Blood was not typed for cattle, so I collected it in open buckets at the time the cattle were killed at the local slaughter house. An anticoagulant was added to the blood at the time of collection. Later the blood was filtered into bottles, dated, and stored in a cool place until used. My father, being of a conservative nature as far as adoption of new methods, did not use blood transfusions. Hindsight indicates he may have been right in his judgment of its effectiveness. However, veterinary science in the late forties indicated its effectiveness. I did, however, encounter an entirely unexpected problem from its use.

Carl Benton was a farmer who lived west of town and raised registered Hereford cattle. He had had occasional cases of yellow fever in past years but this year it struck one pasture in epizootic form. Twenty-four of thirty-two cattle, pastured in one forty-acre pasture, became sick with visible symptoms of the disease. This was an astounding percentage. The only time it was expected to see such percentages was when the ranchers were grossly negligent in the disinfection of dehorning or castration instruments. Carl wasn't guilty of such practices. It could only mean that he had a very effective insect vector operation occurring. One side of the pasture was separated from an adjoining pasture by a tree-shaded fence. His cattle rested under this shade during the heat of the day. Despite frequent spraying, horseflies rested and fed on the cattle at these times. The available insecticide sprays were ineffective against horseflies.

A herd of twenty-five to thirty cattle was in a pasture on the opposite side of the hedge. Another herd of about seventy-five animals was running in a pasture directly across the road from the pasture. To the best of my knowledge, no illnesses resulted in the latter two herds. Horseflies have a formidable set of cutting parts called mandibles attached to their mouth. With these mandibles they are able to slice their way through the hide of cattle and horses so they can suck the blood from such animals. They evidently carried enough blood from infected and carrier animals to the susceptibles in Carl Benton's herd to spread the disease. On the other hand, there could hardly be any doubt but that they also traveled to the other two adjoining herds to feed after feeding on Carl's cattle. Since no disease resulted in these two herds, it indicated that the infectious organism remained viable outside the animal for only a brief period. Apparently, the animals had to be adjacent to each other and only the briefest of time intervals could transpire between bites of the fly vector for it to be possible to transmit the infection. This type of information was valuable at a later date when tests became available to identify the carriers of the infection.

Carl first contacted me the latter part of July. He was busy haying, but he had checked the pasture where the thirty-two head of cattle mentioned previously were running. One heifer seemed to be sluggish and off to itself. Could I come by his house early that evening and pick him up? We would then go on over to the pasture and look at the heifer. Things had been slow during July until then so I was eager to do something.

That evening before dark, Carl and I drove over to the pasture. It was beginning to cool off from the heat of the day so the cattle were out grazing except for one heifer that was lying off by itself. We drove the heifer up into the corner pen, roped, and restrained her. I examined the heifer but noted nothing of significance so treated the animal with penicillin. I advised Carl to watch the heifer and keep me informed, then took him back to his house.

During the next couple of days I was called to see a cow on a farm northwest of New Albany and another on a farm east of Altoona. Both had the distinctive coloration to their mucous membranes that gave the disease its name, "yellow fever." Furthermore, they were anemic and had other symptoms to indicate a diagnosis of anaplasmosis. These cases alerted me to the possibility that the area might be about to experience an anaplasmosis outbreak.

I then received another telephone call from Carl. The heifer didn't seem to be any worse but he had two or three more cattle in the same pasture that were sick. Could I again come by in the early evening after it had begun to cool so we could handle the cattle easier? He would take his horse over in the trailer to help drive the sick cows up to the corner pen where we could handle them easier.

Two of the cows were obviously sick, but they were still "spooky." They tried to break back to the remaining herd when Carl attempted to separate them out to drive up to the catch pen. Even though handled as cautiously as possible, their flanks were heaving by the time they were confined. An examination indicated that they did have anaplasmosis. I treated them supportively but without blood since the demand for blood, until the previous few days, had not existed. I advised Carl of the problem but didn't attempt to sound alarmist since I seldom saw more than two or three cases per farm, although there might be hundreds scattered over the county.

I did go down to one of the local slaughter houses the next day to collect blood for processing. Apparently the anaplasmosis season was at hand so I needed to get prepared. That evening Carl called me back out. One of the cows I had treated the previous day had died. The other one was still sick, but the heifer—the animal I had treated the first day—was apparently better. He had two more sick cows. They were in the pen on arrival. They also had anaplasmosis.

By this time I was becoming alarmed about the situation. Accordingly I gave the sick animals blood transfusions, about 1000 to 2000 ml per animal. This was probably insufficient in quantity but I was trying to ration out the available blood and hoped it might help until I could get more blood.

During the next few days I spent many hours at Carl's, treating cattle with blood transfusions and other medications. It was one of those situations where it seemed like the disease was never going to run its course until all had developed clinical illnesses. Furthermore, the percentage of cattle dying was running at about 25 percent, this in itself an alarming statistic. To top off my concerns, I received a telephone call from Carl one evening. He expressed concern that I was using blood transfusions to treat his cattle. He reminded me that the cattle were "pure bloods." It was probably all right to use blood on ordinary cattle but it was possible that blood lines could be forever compromised by using it in pure bloods. This caught me off guard. I had never imagined a person getting confused about inherited traits being passed through blood rather than the genetic material present in the sperm and ova. I reminded Carl that they transfused blood from one person to another in the hospital without any compromising of genetic traits. Carl reminded me that people were not "pure bloods" like his cattle and restated his concern.

That evening I sat contemplating the possibilities of what Carl had said. That was years before the emergence of genetic engineering as applied science. If Carl was right, and there might be a grain of truth in what he said, it would be possible by means of blood transfusions, judiciously used, to rapidly develop new breeds of cattle and other animals. Furthermore, by treating the blood itself, say with dyes, with sun resisting agents, or with other esoteric substances, people could develop all types of pigmented or tanned skins. Possibly there would be a way to develop zebra stripes on the skin of a temporary nature that could be transfused through the blood at the time of Mardi Gras celebrations. Wouldn't that cause a sensation? My mind was drifting off to still more esoteric ideas—developing better brains, athletic skills, hair and skin color changes, and the like. I would need three parts of this blood and five parts of that blood for this result. Another mix for the other result. As I drifted off to sleep I was beginning to see a whole new field opening up—the field of genetic engineering but using blood products. It might be ahead of its time but . . .

Elsie, the Bloated Cow

"MARIAN, this is Maud."

"Hello, Aunt Maud. How is everybody out there?"

"Fine. Just fine. How are you folks?"

"Oh, I've got a summer cold I can't seem to shake but, except for that, we're all right."

"Those summer colds are the worst ones to get rid of. I had one last summer and didn't shake it until the goldenrod season was over. It might have been one of those hay-fever conditions they talk about. Say, I just called to see if you people would like to come out and eat ice cream. Ote and George are bringing Mrs. Clark, their mother, out. If you can get Sybil and Armer to come, bring them along. I'll call up Lena and see if she and Ed would like to come."

"I'm sure Jim would like to come. I'll telephone Sybil and see if they'll come along."

"Fine. Stop by the ice plant and pick up a hundred pounds of ice and some salt. If we don't use all the ice, I can always put it in the ice box. But, knowing Ote and Junior, I expect we will use it all. They always want to make a second freezer."

"That's all right as long as they turn the crank."

"That was decided years ago. The men turn the crank if they want to eat."

"Well, I'll telephone Sybil and we'll pick up the ice and salt and be out about 6:00 P.M. Is that time all right?"

"Sure. Al may not be through the milking and chores by then but you and Junior can help him."

"Are you sure you have enough cream?"

"I think so—anyway, Ote said he would bring some. They are still milking a couple of cows."

"O.K. then. Thanks for the invitation."

Marian telephoned my mother and she and my father agreed to ride out with us. I came home the latter part of the afternoon and was informed of the plans for the evening. After changing to clean clothes, we drove by and picked up my mother and father, drove by the ice plant and picked up the ice and rock salt, and headed for Aunt Maud and Uncle Al's farm out north of Coyville. We were the first to arrive.

"Al is out at the barn milking the cows. You want to go out and try your hand at it, Marian? My hands have too much arthritis in them to let me grip the teats anymore."

"Sure, I might as well see how he gets the milk. Want to come along, Dad?"

"No, I think I'll stay up here at the house. You and Junior go along."

Marian and I walked down the path to the barnyard gate, opened and closed it as we passed through, and then walked around to the backside of the barn where the door opened into the room with the milking stanchions.

Al and two cows were inside. Two others were awaiting their turns outside. The two inside were confined by their necks in the stanchions. Feed had been placed in the feed box in front of them, and both were eagerly licking up every bit of feed their long protruding tongues could reach. Al was hunched down on a milk stool, two short boards nailed together to form a T. He was supporting a bucket between his knees and had his capped head pressed into the cow's flank. His hands were grasping two of the teats. Rapid squeezing and pulling on the teats was producing two steady streams of milk into the bucket underneath.

"Come on in and grab a bucket. Maud's stool is laying on that bale of hay back behind. She doesn't use it anymore. You might as well use it."

"I don't know how to milk. My fingernails might pinch their teats."

"Squeeze, don't pinch. Go on, get a stool and give it a try."

Marian and I entered the barn. Though hesitant, she gamely walked back and retrieved the stool Al mentioned.

"Can a person really sit on one of these stools?" She tried balancing herself. "It seems like you do a lot of wobbling around."

"That's why you lean up against the cow. It helps you support yourself on the stool. Further, it keeps her off balance so she doesn't crowd you and make you tip over the bucket of milk."

"Well, I'll try. Have you got a cow that's an easy milker. I'm not much of a squeezer."

"That cow in front of you is an easy milker. Besides, she's about dry so won't give much milk. Have Junior put the hobbles on her."

"O.K." After I slipped the hobbles—two V-shaped metal pieces connected by a chain—around her rear legs just above the hocks and pulled the legs together with the chain, Marian crouched down by the cow's flank, stool in one hand, bucket in the other. "Easy, Bossy, nice cow." Marian was putting out her best cow talk trying to soothe the cow now looking back through the stanchion at her.

With one hand she tried to steady the stool while she seated herself on top of the T. With the other hand she tried to steady the bucket between her knees. Her rear end was wobbling, her knees couldn't get a grip on the bucket, the cow shifted her hind legs whenever Marian got near the flank; Marian was perplexed.

"Whoa, cow. Stand still now. Easy." She was trying to console the cow as she edged closer to the flank. It was obvious to her that her knees weren't meant for holding milk buckets so she gingerly slid the bucket underneath the cow's udder while she used two hands to ease her stool and herself closer to the same area. Just as she was about to reach for the teats, the cow, eyeing the situation, decided it was time to act. The cow suddenly shuffled her foot forward and tipped the bucket over. Marian was taken by surprise.

"She doesn't want me to milk her. She kicked the bucket."

"She shoved it, she didn't kick it. If she hadn't been hobbled, you would have known what kicking was. Anyway, that's why you are supposed to hold the bucket between your knees."

"I can't. You hold the bucket while I milk."

She was determined to try. Gamely I crouched ahead of Marian and held the bucket under the cow's udder. "Now go ahead. The cow and I are both waiting."

Marian reached out with one hand and grasped the teat nearest her. She pulled and squeezed. Nothing happened. The cow shifted her rear legs again. "Soo, bossy. I didn't mean to hurt you." Marian carefully put both hands around the teat making certain that her fingernails weren't pinching and squeezed again. This time a thin, short-lived stream appeared—it hardly had enough force to reach the bucket I was holding. "See, I can milk."

"Well, at least that's a start. There's not enough there so far to cover the bottom of the bucket and she's a one-gallon cow, even though nearly dry, according to Uncle Al." When cows aren't giving milk during the month or two before giving birth they are said to be dry.

"That's just the first squirt, here comes the next." This time her two-handed squeeze produced a slightly bigger stream and subsequent squeezing additional streams. "See, I can milk."

"You've got milk all right but she still has three-quarters after this quarter to go. She's not going to wait all night on you."

No sooner had I spoken than the cow shifted the weight on her rear legs and leaned heavily against Marian. Marian, caught off balance, toppled over on her backside. I threw my weight against the cow to protect Marian at the same time holding the milk pail aloft to protect the small quantity of milk contained therein from contamination.

"I don't think she likes me. I'm going up to the house to help Aunt Maud." Saying this, Marian got to her feet, brushed the straw out of her hair and off her clothes, smoothed her dress down, and then without another word, walked out the barn door.

"I don't think we are going to make a milkmaid out of Marian," commented Al, with a smile.

"It was rather a bad introduction," I agreed, grinning back.

"Well, you finish that cow. I'll let Betsy out and put the other two in."

"O.K. They aren't going to get any ice cream mix prepared until we get these cows milked and the cream separated, so we'd better get going."

After we finished the milking and Al let the cows out to pasture for the night, we carried the milk up to the house. Ote, George, their mother, Belle, Lena, and Ed had all arrived.

"Marian said the cows weren't cooperating," Lena said as we opened the door to the screened back porch. "I was about to send Ed down to see if you needed any help."

"I quit milking cows last year when I sold Spot," Ed interjected. "Wouldn't have done any good to send me. I've forgotten how to milk."

"I bet you have. That's what you always say when you don't want to do anything."

"Well, I have. Anyway I'm going into the worm business. Don't have to milk worms to make money," Ed added.

"Tell me about this worm business," demanded Ote. "I'm always looking at new livestock operations. Is it better than fattening calves out?"

"Well, those worms sure don't eat as much as calves do."

"That may be but calves are going for twenty-five dollars per hundred weight on the Wichita market today. What will your worms bring on the market, if there is a market?"

"Harley Jackson is selling them for five cents each or two dollars for a pint-ice-cream container full. I doubt if that container holds a pound of worms," answered Ed.

"Maybe I'd better sell my calves and invest in worms," Ote said.

"That's just when the bottom would drop out of the market," Belle interjected. "It always happens that way. Remember that guinea hen operation?"

"Yes, but . . ." Ote started to reply.

Al had proceeded to start the hand-operated cream separator set in the corner of the back porch. The hum of the separator drowned out the conversation, so the rest of us moved inside the house.

"Junior, grab yourself a piece of chicken off the table before George and Ote eat it all up," Maud advised. "The chicken is what is left over from Al's and my Sunday dinner. We don't hardly eat enough to make it worthwhile to spend the time killing and dressing the chicken. Better eat because it'll be awhile before the ice cream is ready."

"Marian, did you ever pluck a chicken?" Maud was asking.

"No. I think I'll let Jim do the cow milking and chicken plucking in this family," Marian replied.

"When your mother-in-law was engaged to marry Armer, her mother, Lillie, made her learn how to pluck a chicken. Said she would never make a farmer's wife if she couldn't pluck chickens."

"Well, I've never plucked a chicken since we got married," Sybil interrupted. "Armer always dresses the chickens. He took too many chicken disease courses at college and wants to see the insides of the chickens before we eat them."

"Al and I don't know anything about those diseases," laughed Maud. "I guess what we don't know won't hurt us."

By this time I had seated myself at the table and was chewing on the chicken leg. Marian pushed a plate over under my chin. "Jim, if you aren't careful, you'll have food all over Aunt Maud's dinner table."

"Wouldn't cause any problem. It's just oil cloth. Easy to wipe up. Didn't bring out our good linen for you people. You're just family." Maud was hustling in and out of the adjoining kitchen getting things ready for preparing the ice cream mix.

"When the five Porter boys were growing up, Nettie, their sister, used to do the cooking," said Belle Clark. "Nettie had a rule though. She would cook anything they brought in—fish, bird, or animal—but they had to clean it first. Armer and the rest had lots of practice 'cause they sure did like to hunt and fish."

Maud reentered the room from the kitchen at this moment. "Belle, what have you heard from Dora lately?" Dora, Maud and Al's oldest daughter, was married to Guy, one of Belle's sons. "I haven't heard from her in a month's time. She's generally real good about writing."

"Haven't had a letter for about three weeks. She said she was busy at her congressman's Virginia office. Broyhill is running for reelection and it's getting near to election. I expect she'll be tied up until after election. She claims she runs that office. At least she is the only paid employee."

"Expect you're right, Belle. We probably won't see her and Guy until next summer. They don't like to drive out here in the winter."

"She keeps real busy for a person with a medical discharge from civil service," commented Armer wryly.

"You're probably right," said Ote. "Probably never worked half so hard at that job she had with the government as she does now for her Republican congressman."

"Well, she doesn't like it that well. Whenever Guy gets his pension from that bus company, they'll be moving back to Fredonia," commented Belle.

"She might stay if it wasn't for Guy. She is a real politician. Guy, on the other hand, has had his fill of Washington. Been driving buses in the District for twenty years. Says it's getting dangerous to drive at night because of robberies. He refuses to drive at night—guess he's got enough seniority to get away with it," Ote explained.

"Well, I worked back in Washington when I first graduated from college," Marian said. "Sixty days was enough for me. I was a young bride and went back to live with Jim during his last year in college. I was hired as a dietitian in one of those government cafeterias. All I did was try to get a crew of lazy people to keep the place clean. Never cooked a potato while I was there."

"Been cheaper to contract that work out," said Armer. "Wouldn't have to end up pensioning all those people off." He was always the practical minded person, especially when it came to money.

Just then the telephone rang—two shorts and a long. "That's our ring." Maud crossed the room to the wall-mounted telephone. "Hello," she spoke into the receiver after lifting the ear piece off its hook and holding it to her ear.

"Oh, hello, Mabel." After a pause, "Yes, it certainly has been a scorcher. We're fixing to make ice cream. Thought maybe it would cool us off." Another pause. "Yes, Junior and Armer are both here—

how did you know?" Mabel was the operator at the Coyville telephone exchange. She knew everything but it was always polite to ask. "Well, that's what they pay you telephone operators for, isn't it?" Another pause. "Don't get much pay. I guess none of us do. Who do you want, Junior or Armer?"

"Junior," Maud turned to me, "Mabel up at the telephone office tracked you down. Heard me talking to Marian this afternoon. Hank Broderick, up the road, needs a vet fast. He'll take either Armer or you. His wife, Helen, is on the line."

"Damn," I muttered under my breath. "Can't get away from the telephone." I laid the chicken bone on which I was gnawing on the plate, looked over at my father, shook my head, arose, and crossed over to the telephone. Armer just smiled. He had been through it for many years by himself before I returned to practice.

Maud handed the receiver to me. "Hello, this is Jim Porter. What's your trouble?" A pause. "Bloated. Tell Hank I'll be right there. She's there at your barn just up the road from here at Al's place, right?" I put the receiver back on the hook and turned and smiled wanly at my father. "Hank Broderick has a bloated cow. I presume you want me to do the honors."

"Why not? I'll stay here and see that Ote doesn't eat up all the ice cream."

"Who's going to watch you?" Ote asked. "Besides, we can always make a second freezer."

"I didn't know there was any 'can' about it," Maud said. "When haven't we made that second freezer?"

"Well, I'll go with Junior," Ed volunteered. "If I stay here, I'll have to turn the crank."

"You really have retired since you started getting that social security check, haven't you?" Lena was chiding Ed again. He grinned. He hadn't gotten the last word in since Lena said "I do" at their wedding.

Ed and I walked out to my station wagon and got inside. I started the motor, backed out of the yard, and drove the mile up the road to the Broderick's. As a veterinary practitioner, I used the station wagon for dual purposes and never unloaded it since I never knew when I might need my equipment and drugs. When we drove into Broderick's yard, we saw Helen frantically waving her arms out by the barn motioning us to hurry.

"Hank's around behind the barn. Hurry! Hurry! Elsie's about dead."

I jumped out of the car, ran through the barn door held open by

Helen and emerged from the other side of the barn through another open door. There was Elsie stretched out on her side, head extended, tongue protruded with her eyes rolled back in her head. Her left flank was gashed open and a green frothy material alternately spewed and spouted from the opening. The frothy material collected on either side where it ran off her sides. She was panting and gasping for breath. The whole area smelled strongly of methane gas. To make the scene more bizarre, Hank stood over Elsie, knife in one raised hand, while the other hand frantically tried to scoop the spewing froth out of the open paunch.

"What the hell are you trying to do, Hank? Get her up on her belly or she is going to die on you."

"Hell, she would have been dead if I hadn't cut her open," replied Hank. "She was about ready to float away with all that gas in her—dead or not dead."

While he was talking the four of us managed to prop Elsie's front legs back under her and roll her upon her sternum. Elsie raised her head slightly and let out a belch that spewed greenish froth for six feet or more in front of her, barely missing Helen. "God, she stinks. I sure don't want to get that on me." Helen grimaced. The front of Hank's clothes from head to toe was covered with the froth. Whenever the material spouted, Hank caught the full force of it.

"I don't care what I smell like. I just want to keep her alive. We sure can't afford to start buying milk." Hank was still desperately scooping the material out of the exposed paunch. The spume formed as fast as he could get it out of her. Ruminants have a four compartment stomach. The first compartment is called the paunch or rumen and is used as a fermentation vat to break down the roughages consumed into usable nutrients. Some roughages at certain growth stages produce fermentation and gas formation faster than ruminants can belch the gas up, thus resulting in bloat. The treatment is to pass a stomach tube or pierce the bloated paunch to relieve the pressure and prevent death.

"Where did you learn to start operating on cows that way?" I asked.

"My daddy taught me this years ago but I think I was a little over zealous with this cut. I was scared. She looked like she was dying."

"Overzealous and then some. That gash is a foot and a half long."

"Doc, do something! I didn't call you up here to critique my surgery."

"You're doing great, Hank. I'll get some medicine from the station wagon and see if we can't stop that gas from forming."

I returned a few minutes later with a pail containing an antibloat medicine and a stomach tube. In place of running the tube through the mouth, down the throat, and into the paunch, I attached one end of the tube to the pump sticking out of the pail and inserted the other end directly into the paunch. Ed manned the pump while I tried to move my end of the tube into and around the depths of the paunch. Elsie continued to alternately spew and spout the greenish spume through the gapping wound in her flank. As soon as I joined Hank over that eruptive area, I was met by an explosion of that odorous material. My face, hair, neck, and shirt were covered by the greenish froth. It filled my nostrils, ears, eyes, and, when I opened it, my mouth. I stank and was filthy.

"Join the crowd," Hank invited. "Now let's get to work."

"Junior, you're going to have to get a longer hose or find another pumper," Ed complained. "That gunk is piling up by my feet. I don't like the smell or the looks of it and I know Lena's not going to let me back into the house if I get that stuff on me."

"I'm not sure Marian is going to accept me either," I replied. "Finish pumping that medicine in that bucket and then back up. Hank and I will handle it. Won't we, Hank?"

"I hope it's we. That's what I got you here for, Doc."

"What in the world did she bloat on, Hank?" I inquired.

"Somebody left the gate down. She got into the alfalfa field. It was lush from last Wednesday's rain."

"It really made a brewery out of her paunch. Too bad people don't have a taste for this stuff. We could bottle it and sell it."

"I wish we could. Helen, why don't you take this knife. I don't think I'm going to do any more cutting and Doc may start getting nervous with me waving this knife around."

"I think you've done enough cutting," I agreed. "Let's get her emptied out and sewn up."

I returned to my station wagon to get a supply of suture material and the accompanying supplies to anesthetize, clean, and dress the area.

"How you doing, Hank? Gaining on her?" I inquired when I returned.

Hank was still raking the froth out, this time with both hands. He didn't reply and his face was covered with slime so I couldn't tell whether he was smiling or frowning at developments.

Elsie let out another belch, spewing the froth in front of her.

"Look, Elsie is trying to help you out," Helen said encouragingly.

Elsie seemed to confirm Helen's words when she looked back at Hank and me and let out a "Moooo . . ." She didn't have too much volume to it but she was trying to communicate.

"That looks better. What did you pump into her? That might be good for that indigestion I get after some of Helen's suppers."

"Another comment like that, Mr. Broderick, and Mrs. Broderick is not going to cook any more suppers for Mr. Broderick."

"I'm sorry, Helen. I was all wrapped up in my work and wasn't thinking."

"I don't know about being wrapped up in your work but you're certainly knee deep in it."

"Hank, we seem to be gaining on the bloat. Let me throw some 'stay' stitches in that paunch so we can keep that abdominal cavity from getting contaminated. She was so bloated when you sliced her open that the paunch stuck out through her incised hide. As the pressure eases, the paunch is going to start receding and that gunk is going to start leaking inside."

I proceeded to insert the 'stay' stitches to keep the paunch anchored outside. Next, with Hank still scooping and me dodging the spewing slime, I started suturing from the bottom. I was supposed to suture the hide, the external muscles, the peritoneum, and the paunch separately. I'm certain that my surgery professor, Dr. E. R. Frank, would never have approved of the job I did. Barnyard surgery is a field unto itself. However, I did manage to get the layers back together although there may not always have been the clear separation of muscle and peritoneal layers. A couple of hours later Elsie was back in one piece and I had left Hank a trocar with instructions for its use. A trocar is a large metal canula with a sharp-pointed instrument within. After using the pointed instrument to pierce the flank, that instrument is removed and the canula left in the paunch to serve as a vent for the gas. "This trocar only leaves a one-half inch opening," I told Hank. "You don't have to sew up the wound when you extract the trocar; besides I don't think your daddy taught you to make an eighteen-inch bloat incision. He wouldn't have done it over once. You got carried away."

"I was scared," answered Hank. "I really thought Elsie was dying and I was just trying to get that stuff out. Doc, come on up to the back porch and let's get cleaned up."

"That's a good idea except I think I need a change of clothes."

"You'd better. The inside of that car is never going to smell the same if you try to drive in those clothes," Ed advised me.

"I'll get you a change of clothes," volunteered Helen. "You and Hank are about the same size. You can strip off those clothes, shower, and dress in some of Hank's clothes. I'll bring in your washed clothes the next time we come to Fredonia and we can pick up Hank's then."

It sounded like a practical idea. Helen preceded us to the house to find some clean clothes, soap, and towels. Hank and I stopped on the boardwalk that ran from the back door to the outside well. It was now dark so Hank and I stripped off our clothes and stood naked on the walk. "I won't look," shouted Helen. "Ed can bring out the clean clothes, soap, and towels."

"This ought to be fun," chuckled Ed.

"You don't know the half of it, Ed," laughed Hank. "You're going to have the honor of drawing up the water bucket from that well and dousing us while Doc and I soap ourselves down."

"I knew I was going to get caught somehow," Ed said. "Well, I suppose Helen is too modest to douse Junior down and we did have ice cream waiting down at Al's so let's get started."

"Helen is not modest but Doc might be, even in the dark," said Hank. I figured I'd better not try replying to that. In the darkness, Ed drew up the water pails from the well and poured the water over us. Hank and I soaped, rinsed, toweled ourselves, and dressed in clean clothes.

When Ed and I started to leave, Hank called out, "We'll leave a check when we bring your clothes in. Thanks for saving Elsie's life."

As we drove back to Al's, Ed inquired, "Junior, it's none of my business, but what are you going to charge Hank?"

"I was wondering that myself. What would Dr. Bill Jones charge if he did that surgery repair up at St. Margaret's Hospital?"

"More than Elsie is worth, I'll bet."

"I think you're right."

We had arrived at Al's and rejoined the others.

"What kept you so long?" asked Marian. "We are just opening up the second freezer."

"You tell her, Ed," I replied.

"It's like I said when we left," explained Ed. "If we had returned sooner, I'd had to turn the crank on the freezer."

I shrugged as Aunt Maud handed me the first dish of ice cream scooped out of the opened freezer. Only my father could have understood, so why try to elaborate on Ed's explanation.

The Card Game

"MARIAN, I just called to see if you and Doc would like to come over and play bridge tonight?" Betsy Brown was on the line. "Bob says he feels lucky and that he and Doc are going to wipe up on us to get even for last week's fiasco."

"We did have some good cards, didn't we," Marian replied. "Let me ask Jim. He's lying down on the couch listening to the news."

"No wonder he's so smart. The only thing Bob listens to is sports. He won't even read the newspaper headlines unless it's about a murder or a sex crime."

"Can't get the cop out of him, can you? Hold the line, let me ask Jim."

A few minutes later Marian was back on the line. "We'll be over about 7:30. Jim says he feels lucky too."

"They need a few more lessons from us, don't they? It takes more than luck at bridge." Betsy was speaking confidently. "I'll see if I can get Joey tucked in for the night before you get here."

"That'll be the time—anyway, he won't bother us. Just give him some crayons and a color book. That should keep him busy."

"You're optimistic, aren't you? We'll be looking for you about 7:30. I'm still going to try to get Joey down before you get here. He can be a nuisance trying to grab cards from my hand and off the table."

"Can I bring anything, Betsy?" Marian asked.

"No, of course not. I'll just whip up a little something for dessert before we finish the last game."

"Those little somethings are putting the pounds on Bob and Jim. Their stomachs are hanging out over their belts just like Tex Malone, Chuck Stewart, and some of those other cattlemen who come into Jim's office."

"They do look a little pregnant, don't they? Well, they say the way to a man's heart is through his stomach. We sure wouldn't want them to get roaming eyes, would we?"

"We'll see you at 7:30," replied Marian as she hung up.

At 7:30 we knocked on the door of the Brown's house. A yell was heard from within, "Mommy, mommy, door."

"I hear it, Joey. It's probably the Porters. Can you open the door and let them in? No, let me help you. It's locked and you won't be able to open it." We could hear feet running toward the door. A few seconds later we heard the lock being released and the door opened to admit us. "Come on in you two. Now Joey, let go of Marian's skirt. She can't move with you hanging all over her." Betsy, a buxom lady with an infectious good nature, lightly slapped Joey's hands.

"He's all right. Just glad to see me, aren't you, Joey?" asked Marian as she unfastened Joey's hands from her skirt. "My, you're getting big. How old are you now?"

"Almost two, aren't you Joey? When are you and Doc going to get started? How long have you been married now?" Betsy was always trying to be helpful.

"Going on four years. We're trying. Maybe Jim is going to have to get some inside information from Bob."

"Maybe I should loan you Bob for a night or two. I think he could handle a harem," volunteered Betsy.

"Thanks, but no thanks. I'll just let nature take its course. Besides, Dr. Adams did that tubal procedure on me last year and says I can't get pregnant."

"Adopt a baby—you'll get pregnant."

"That does seem to happen, doesn't it?"

I was a little embarrassed by the conversation so slipped by the ladies into the living room. "Besty, where's Bob?" I inquired.

"Oh, he's finishing his bath. He'll be out in a minute. Got home late from the shop so didn't bathe before eating. He was dirty and smelly. He needed the bath."

Just then, as on cue, Bob emerged from the bedroom, a big grin on his face. He was a large man, six foot one or two, and weighed well over two hundred pounds. His weight, as mine, was not as well distributed as it should have been. It tended to mass in the stomach area and hang out as a roll of fat over his belt. "Doc, come give me a belly bump." After bumping bellies he said, "I don't think you've lost any weight over the weekend. Marian must still be feeding you."

"You two are a mess. You both should go on a diet," said Betsy.

"Then we wouldn't be able to bump bellies. You wouldn't want us to go back to shaking hands, would you?" asked Bob. "Besides, you keep serving those midnight snacks."

"That's to put you to sleep, my dear," replied Betsy. "If I didn't do that I might never get to sleep."

"Always complaining," explained Bob. "Is Marian like that, Doc?"

"I'd better not answer that."

"To return to the belly bumping, that isn't particularly attractive. Shaking hands would be a lot more esthetic," said Marian.

Just then the phone rang. Betsy picked it up. "Hello." A pause. "Yes, this is the Brown's residence." Another pause. "Sure is. Let me call him."

"Doc, it's for you." Betsy handed me the phone. "Can't get away from the telephone, can he, Marian?"

"The operators do seem to track him down. He transfers his calls when he goes out. Real inconvenient sometimes," added Marian.

"Hello. Yes, this is Dr. Porter. What can I do for you?" A pause. "No, I don't have office hours at night. You'll have to bring Mitzie into the office during the day to get her the rabies shot." A pause. "Yes, I know Armer vaccinated dogs at night but he worked out of his house. I don't have an office at my house. Give me a ring when you have some extra time in the next day or two. I'm sure you'll catch me in sometime." Another pause. "O.K., I'll see you then. Tell Mitzie to relax for the evening." I put down the phone.

"You got out of that one, didn't you, Doc?" observed Bob. "Maybe you should bring your vaccine with you and vaccinate dogs over here. You could use the kitchen table. Betsy wouldn't charge you much for the use of the table, would you, Betsy?"

"We never would get any cards played if I started doing that."

"Come on. Sit down. I've got the decks out. Let's play." Betsy was impatiently shuffling cards.

Bob and I took chairs opposite each other. Marian and Betsy were already seated. "Draw for deal."

Just then the phone rang again. "It's going to be one of those nights," I commented.

"Yes, he's here." Betsy had answered the phone. "It's for you, Doc."

"You get the phone, Doc. I'll watch to see that they don't stack the deck on us."

I shook my head, arose, and walked over and took the phone from Betsy.

"Hello." A pause. "Yes, this is Junior." Another pause. "Just getting set to play cards." Another pause. "No, we don't gamble. I don't think Sheriff Jackson would be interested in this game. What can I do for you?" Another pause. "Rabies, yes, cows do have rabies, but I doubt if she has rabies." Another pause. "You say she's bloated?

Now that begins to add up." Another pause. "Yes, I'll be right out." I put down the phone and turned to my companions waiting at the table.

"That was Elmer Burton out east of town. He's got a bloated cow so I'd better go. Want to come along, Bob?"

"Sure, why not? Keep those cards warm for us while we're away."

Bob got up from his chair and joined me going out the door.

About ten minutes later we drove into the Burton's driveway and saw a lantern directing us on out toward the barn.

"Sure glad you could come out, Junior. Jersey is all bloated up. Getting bigger all the time."

"She needs some attention. Glad I could come."

"Come on in and take a look."

I followed Elmer into the barn and back to the stanchion where Jersey was confined. Elmer was a wizened old man with a weathered face and calloused hands brought on by years of farm work. He was joined by his son-in-law, George Evans, who lived at the adjoining farm. George, though younger, was just the opposite of Elmer. He was heavy, his face was full and relatively unwrinkled, and his hands were smooth. He worked in town at a local filling station pumping gas and rented out his farm land.

"What do you think?" inquired George. "Does she have rabies?"

"Where do you get this rabies stuff? She's bloated."

"But she sure was slobbering earlier this evening and she couldn't drink water. Those are symptoms of rabies, aren't they?"

"They can be symptoms of something else, too," I replied. "Wait a minute until I get some tools from the car." I left Bob with the two men and returned to my station wagon.

"Junior bringing you along to learn the business, is he?" inquired Elmer.

"I don't think so. My stomach couldn't take some of those rotten afterbirth jobs," responded Bob.

"You served in the Marines in the South Pacific, didn't you?" asked George. "I heard some of those dead Japs got to stinking."

"I spent some time out there with the 'gyrenes' on Guadalcanal. I don't know if you call that serving or not. Actually, I didn't see too many dead Japs. They would retrieve the bodies after their night attacks if they could. Didn't want us to run body counts."

"I understand Hal Hughes was was out there with you," said George.

"He sure was. We were foxhole buddies many a night out on the perimeter line."

"I'll bet that was scary."

"It was. I remember the night a rat jumped in the foxhole with me. Thought it was a Jap for a minute. I think I dirtied my underpants a little that night. It was scary."

"You and Hal both came through all right, didn't you?" asked George.

"Luckily yes."

I returned with a few pieces of equipment. After adjusting a wooden mouth gag in Jersey's mouth, I slipped a two-inch stiff hose through the central opening in the mouth gag. After some manipulation I passed it into and down the esophagus. Before entering the rumen, it met an obstacle.

"There's your trouble. She's choked!" I said.

"Choked! Can't be! What could she get choked on?" asked Elmer.

"Look." I applied a little pressure to the tube and the obstructing body was pushed on into the rumen. Immediately a rush of gas released by the freeing of the esophageal obstruction was emitted from the tube.

"That stinks," said Bob, holding his nose closed with his fingers. "Did you do something, George?"

"Don't look at me, Bob," countered George. "Look at Jersey's flank. That bloat is going down fast."

As George had pointed out, the bloat was indeed being reduced by the passage of the accumulated gas through the stomach tube to the exterior.

"I guess you made a believer out of me, Junior, but what did she get choked on?" again asked Elmer.

"I don't know but I expect it was on a piece of one of those hedge apples that are lying underneath your hedge trees. The cows think they are a delicacy and tend to swallow them in big chunks rather than chewing them up. Sometimes those chunks are just too large to pass through the restriction caused by the diaphragm," I explained.

After putting my tools back into the station wagon and collecting a check and thanks from Elmer, Bob and I returned to Bob's house.

As we entered, Bob shouted ahead, "Get those cards shuffled, we're ready to go."

"Not tonight, Bob. Doc's got another call," explained Betsy.

"Another call? What's it this time?" Bob was unhappy.

"It is important. Jack Lambert has a cow calving and needs some assistance," said Marian.

"You two do sit down. I have a cake just coming out of the oven. Doc has to eat a piece before going on, don't you, Doc?"

"I guess I could use some refreshment. Bob, we're just going to have to put that card game off until another night."

"I think I would be lucky tomorrow night. What do you say to taking a 'rain check' until then?" asked Bob.

We agreed that would be satisfactory. After the cake and a cup of coffee, we excused ourselves and I dropped Marian off at the house before driving out to Jack Lambert's.

Two hours later I slipped into bed beside Marian.

"What took you so long? Jack just lives a couple of miles south, doesn't he?"

"The calf's head was turned back. My arms are really sore from working inside that cow."

"Well, you can sleep a little later in the morning."

"Not hardly. The signs are right so I have to be at Jeff Lincoln's to work his calves. They'll be ready by 8:30 A.M., so this is going to be a short night."

Thirty seconds later I was fast asleep.

Gwendolyn Gets Hooked

I was sitting in church with my wife on a warm July Sunday. The doors and windows were wide open. Overhead fans were lazily stirring the air around the room. Most of the parishioners were fanning themselves with fans donated by the Cason Funeral Home. The other parishioners were nodding their heads. Reverend A. C. Martin, minister of our congregation, was in full form. Sweat was pouring off his brow (he had a high forehead—in fact, only a fringe of hair remained) as he exhorted the congregation with sweeping gestures of his arms interspersed with pulpit pounding to repent of their sins and prepare for salvation. Reverend Martin had been converted as a youth at a tent revival meeting in Kansas City. The fervor of that meeting had rubbed off on him. He was a natural revival speaker, casting devils out and bringing souls to salvation. He would probably have followed the revival circuit except that he had a wife and two sons and needed to establish roots someplace so he could raise his sons. The Christian church in Fredonia was blessed with his services for some twenty years.

Reverend Martin approached every sermon with the premise that there were those in the audience who needed to be saved and this was the Sunday he would successfully plead with them to come forward, confess their sins, and join in the great Army of the Lord. The only problem was that all in the audience were already members except for the children, and Easter was the time of the year the children came forward to unite with Christ. But in those days people weren't able to turn on their television sets on Sunday and hear the great revivalists. They had a revivalist in their pulpit, and they turned out in good numbers Sunday after Sunday to see our preacher give battle with Satan.

"Yes, the Lord first tempted man when he sent the serpent to Eve to inveigle her to taste of the forbidden fruit—and he is tempting you and me every day with forbidden fruit—are we weak like Eve or are we strong . . . ?"

I was being nudged by Marian. I turned and she pointed to the aisle. The usher was motioning to me. I arose and squeezed my way from my seat past the other persons sitting between me and the aisle. In some cases there just wasn't leg room and the person had to stand up to allow my passage. This was causing considerable commotion, so

Reverend Martin ceased his orating. I had interrupted him at the critical point in his sermon but there was nothing he could do until I was out of the building. He mopped the sweat off his forehead with a large white handkerchief he carried in his coat pocket for just that purpose. My face reddened, realizing I was the object of every eye in the room. Those who were asleep had been awakened by my exit. I tried to shrink as much as possible as I walked up the aisle and out of the church with the usher. As I walked out the door I heard the preacher cough loudly a couple of times—and then relaunch his exhortation of the congregation.

Waiting outside was Si Peterson. "Junior, I'm sure sorry to bother you but Gwendolyn is in trouble."

"Who's Gwendolyn, and what's happened, Si?" I had already put the church service out of my mind.

"Gwendolyn is my wife's duck. If anything happens to her, my wife will banish me to sleeping on the couch. Gwendolyn has swallowed a fish hook. She's over there in my car."

My mind began functioning on what was to be done. "Si, I'll leave my car here for my wife, and you can drive me and Gwendolyn down to my office where we'll see what can be done."

I slipped into the front seat of the car with Si. Gwendolyn was in a small cage on the back seat. "O.K., let's go."

A few minutes later we arrived at my office. I unlocked the door and Si carried the cage inside and put it on the examining table. "Now tell me what happened." We had visited about the weather on the trip to the office—ten days in a row with over one-hundred-degree temperatures—and about the crops—the wheat was turning out good but the corn could certainly use some rain. I now needed to find out what had caused me to miss the last part of the preacher's fight with the devil.

"Well, Lucille, that's my wife, she went to church this morning. I'm not much for church going, you know. It being a nice day and nothing pressing to do in the fields, I decided to go down to the creek and try out that fishing reel my son gave me for a birthday present. My son's working up in Wichita helping build planes for Cessna now. Not enough work to keep him down on the farm. Anyway, I picked up the reel and tackle box and headed for the creek. It's about a quarter mile away. Gwendolyn, she follows right along behind me. She's a pet, you know, given to Lucille when just a duckling and raised by hand. Wouldn't know what another duck was, she wouldn't.

Well, anyway we got to the creek and Gwendolyn dove right in and started swimming around while I was getting my fishing gear ready. A few minutes later I had a lure attached to the line on my reel and cast it out toward the water. That dumb Gwendolyn thought is was some kind of fly, I guess. She scooted over that water and grabbed that lure before it could hit the water. Swallowed it hook, line, and sinker. Well, not really. She did swallow the lure and hook though."

By this time I had Gwendolyn out of her cage and was examining the situation. She had indeed swallowed the hook and lure. The hook was lodged somewhere in the pharyngeal region. "I'd have taken it out myself if it had been a fish, but being Lucille's pet duck I was afraid to try it. It would be my luck to kill the duck and then my banishment to the couch. What can you do, Junior?"

"You lend me a hand and we'll get Gwendolyn fixed up so you can keep sleeping with Lucille."

"I sure hope so. What can I do?"

"You use this instrument to keep her bill pried open. I'll see what I can do with the hook."

An examination revealed that the barb of the hook had penetrated the pharyngeal wall. The point was just under the skin. "May not be too bad. You just hold Gwendolyn still and keep that mouth pried open."

"All right, but don't tear her up too much inside. She's got to live if I'm to stay out of the doghouse for letting her go to the creek with me."

"I won't tear her up any more than already done." Saying this, I managed to grasp the shank of the hook with a clamp and force the point to the outside. After the point had penetrated the skin, I cut it off with a set of dikes and easily removed the barbless hook back through the mouth. Si was in ecstasy. "You did it, Junior. You did it. I've always told my neighbors you were every bit as good as Armer and now you sure proved it."

Gwendolyn expressed her gratitude at having the hook removed and being released from the manhandling, by ruffling up her feathers, stretching her legs, quacking a couple of times, and then depositing a big dropping on the table. "That's her way of saying thank you, Junior. Here, let me clean it up. Lucille doesn't let her get up on the table out at the farm. She's just not table trained."

Sometime later, Si let me off at my home. When I entered, Marian asked me what was so important that I had to interrupt the church service and embarrass her. After I explained to her, she just shook her head.

"Your mother would say, that's the Lord's punishment to Si Peterson for violating the Sabbath."

"But it was Gwendolyn, not Si, who got hooked."

"Just as she would say, that's what happens when you violate the Sabbath."

She had my mother and the Lord on her side so I ceased arguing. "If I don't have any more calls to violate the Sabbath with, I think I'll read the Sunday paper while you get dinner on the table."

"I've yet to see the Sunday when you don't have calls. Dinner will be on the table shortly."

The telephone rang. I laid down the newspaper and walked over to the telephone. As Marian had said, Sunday was just another working day for me.

The Turtle Vets

SYBIL, is Armer there?"

"No, who's calling?"

"This is Chuck Baxter. I've got a turtle to sell him."

My father ate turtle meat. While turtle meat is considered a delicacy in many areas, it and opposum were considered unfit for decent people to eat in rural Kansas. My mother never would adjust her sensitivity enough to prepare the turtle. Armer dressed and cooked turtle. My mother, with my sisters and myself, did eat the meat. We all agreed it was good as prepared by my father.

Father used to pick up large turtles he would see on the roadside as he traveled about his practice. After the word spread that Armer ate turtle, people would bring turtles to him. Still, in later years, people attempted to sell him turtles they collected in the country. He refused to start buying turtles, but the calls persisted.

"Armer doesn't buy turtles."

"I know, but this one is eighteen inches across. He'll want to buy this one."

"No, he won't."

"Now, Sybil, you ask Armer."

"He doesn't buy turtles."

"Sybil, this turtle is badly hurt. I can't turn it loose."

"Well, bring it in. Maybe Armer will look at it."

"He won't charge me, will he? I guess I'll give him the turtle but I can't afford to pay any veterinary bill on it."

"I guess he hasn't started charging for doctoring turtles yet. O.K., bring the turtle by."

A couple of hours later, Chuck showed up at the back door carrying a large turtle with a badly damaged carapace (shell). Evidently it had been run over by a car. It hadn't been killed, but the carapace was split open the full length of the shell.

"Leave him in the washtub there by the hydrant. I'll tell Armer when he gets back."

When Armer returned, Sybil informed him of the call and the donation of another turtle.

"Armer, where do these people get the idea that you buy turtles? It's disgusting."

"Sybil, I don't buy turtles. You do like eating the meat so it must not be too disgusting."

"There's one in the washtub I'm not eating. It's been hurt."

"Let's take a look."

After examining the turtle, Armer agreed that it wouldn't be wise to eat an injured turtle. We might get sick.

"I'll go ahead and kill it."

"No, you can't do that, Armer." Mother had suddenly developed a compassionate feeling for the turtle. "Can't you put him back together?"

"Sybil, why in the world would I want to do that?"

"Because I asked you to."

That was sufficient reason. Later that afternoon when I got home, Marian told me I had a call from my father. He wanted me to come over.

"O.K. You want to come along?"

"No. You go along. I'll get supper ready."

When I arrived at my parents' home, Armer took me around to the back to look at the turtle.

"Junior, did you ever work on a turtle at college?"

"No."

"Well, we're going to work on one now. Your mother isn't going to give me any peace until I do something."

"All right. Let's see what we can do."

An examination revealed no serious internal injuries. We drilled two-inch holes parallel on each side of the split in the carapace and threaded wire through the holes. We then pulled the shell together. Before tying the wires together, we glued a piece of canvas over the rejoined area. We then tied the two ends of each wire together after pulling them snug.

"You're now an experienced turtle veterinarian. I'll send my turtle cases to you, Junior."

"No, thank you. I think it would be 'pro gratis' work. You can have it if you want it."

"I think I'd rather kill and dress them than put them back together."

"How are you going to keep the turtle? Mother won't let you keep it on the back porch and it can escape under the garage door."

"I'll fix a pen in the back yard. I've never fattened turtles out to eat. Guess there's always a first time."

Accordingly, he constructed a pen in the backyard from a few stakes and a roll of poultry wire. The turtle made a remarkable recovery. It would move around the pen eating grass and the lettuce, berries, and other fruit and vegetable scraps that my father fed it.

"That's going to be mighty expensive turtle meat," he told me one day. "Considering the surgery, time, and food I've got in it, it's probably worth five dollars a pound."

"That is expensive. When are you going to kill it?"

"What about this week? Marian and you come over next Sunday and we'll eat turtle."

"We'll look forward to it."

The next Sunday Marian and I showed up for dinner and Mother served roast beef and potatoes. I said nothing but after dinner when we were in the front room, I asked my father what had occurred.

"Sybil wouldn't let me kill it. All the 4-H kids sell their stock at auction after the fair. That's the reason for fattening livestock, but Sybil wouldn't agree. She had named that turtle 'Slowpoke' and had become attached to it. Said she'd never eat Slowpoke. She never would be a livestock raiser. I had to release the turtle out in the country."

"I guess you don't need to plan on fattening out a hog then. Mother would make you release it too."

Father just shook his head and changed the subject.

"I'm Trading Two $10,000 Cows for a $20,000 Bull"

FREDONIA was buzzing with rumors. The Campbells were moving their Polled Hereford operation from Texas to Fredonia. Tom Campbell had made Clinton, Texas, world famous as the home of his Polled Hereford herd that had won more than its share of blue ribbons at the various cattle shows over the country. Now Fredonia was to have this reflected glory as the home of this famous herd. The ranch at Clinton had been taken over by the Corps of Engineers to make way for the Big Webster Dam. Tom Campbell was retiring and turning the herd over to his son, Frank. It was reported that they had selected Fredonia as the new home for their herd because of its location central to the market and because of its friendly people. At least the local chamber of commerce promoted the idea of the friendly people. The probability was that the land was priced right.

I'm certain the feed dealers, the gasoline supply men, the insurance agents, and representatives of most other businesses had stopped at the Campbells soliciting business. Rumors continued to spread after each of these visits about the future the Campbells had planned for their Fredonia operation. I awaited developments. Veterinarians in those days considered it unethical to solicit business. Besides, my father and I were the only veterinarians for thirty to forty-five miles around Fredonia. I presumed we would eventually be approached by the Campbells. I was used to working on cattle that had a value of $100 to possibly $500 a head. I did wonder what it would be like to be working on cattle that were reported to be worth thousands of dollars each.

One day the call came. I drove out to the ranch. One of the bull calves in the show barn was bloated. Some medicine pumped into the paunch of the calf, some exercise, and some tincture of time relieved the situation. It also opened up a professional association that was to last for several years.

"Dr. Porter, the secret of a successful cattle operation is to develop a reputation by showing cattle and to have periodic auction sales to capitalize on one's reputation."

This sounded reasonable. I had worked with the Charles McGraw

Angus herd and with the herd of his nephew, Steve. Charles McGraw had in previous years shown cattle and developed a reputation. He was now living on his reputation and selling cattle directly from his ranch to individual buyers. Steve McGraw would develop a reputation as a showman and as a seller of quality Angus. At that time nobody in the area was conducting the type of operation that the Campbells were proposing and certainly nobody claimed they had cattle that would equal the quality claimed for the stock on the Campbell ranch.

Frank Campbell continued his explanation. "Dad made a killing on the dispersal sale he held after the government bought our land—only it wasn't a complete dispersal. I've got many of the foundation animals here to start rebuilding with. I'm bringing in Rex Domino 167 to be my primary herd sire. Rex Domino won the '59 Grand Championship at Chicago and was runner-up at Kansas City the same year. He is out of Rex Domino 112, who won more ribbons than any other bull ever has. Yes sir, you've got to plan these things. I'm getting Rex Domino for $20,000. That is more money than was ever paid for any bull that ever set foot in this county."

"That sure is a lot of money Mr. Campbell."

"Well, I don't actually have that much money tied up in him. I'm trading two cows worth $5,000 each and a couple of future heifer picks for the bull. When you operate at our level you don't actually deal in cash."

"Then how do you know the cows are worth $5,000 each? If they were worth only $2,500 each, the bull wouldn't be worth as much."

Frank Campbell grimaced at my suggestion. "I see I've got a lot to teach you, Dr. Porter. When I have my sale here, I'll have buyers from all over the United States and cattle will average $5,000 each."

"Well, I've got a lot to learn. I'll certainly be mighty interested in seeing cattle sell for $5,000 each."

"Incidentally, Dr. Porter, I'll need you to fill out the health papers on Rex Domino 167. I'm insuring him with Hartford."

"Of course, Mr. Campbell. Whenever you get the papers I'll be happy to make the examination."

"Now, Dr. Porter, I'll be needing your help from time to time. These cattle are in a class above the cattle you deal with around here, but I'm certain we can make out."

"Thank you, Mr. Campbell, I think I may be able to manage."

"Dr. Porter, what I'm aiming for now is to have a sale in a couple of years. I want it right after the American Royal in Kansas City when a lot of the big buyers will be in this part of the country. Yes sir, I'm going to plan it right and make a fortune on that sale."

"Well, at $5,000 a head, that will amount to a lot of money. I wish you well."

We shook hands and I drove back to my office.

One day the report circulated that Frank Campbell had lost a $2,000 cow. It seemed that the cow had stuck its head through a barbed wire fence, and while attempting to withdraw her head, she had entangled the neck chain to which her metal identification tag was attached in the wire. In the ensuing struggle to free herself, she had managed to lose her footing. When found, she was dead either from asphyxiation or bloat or both. The stockmen in the area clucked their tongues knowingly. Anybody who would be so highfalutin as to have neck chains for cattle deserved to lose them. No self-respecting cattleman in the area would consider using any identification other than a hot iron brand or, in the case of registered cattle, a tattoo in the ear. Campbell would learn.

One of the next encounters I had with the Campbell herd was when Frank Campbell called me in for consultation. His cows weren't settling; that is they were coming back into heat repeatedly even though a bull was running in the pasture with them.

"Dr. Porter, Domino Star 23rd isn't settling the cows he's running with over in the west pasture. I need to get those cows bred now so they'll calf in time to be bred back to Red Domino 167 before the sale time."

"Well, Mr. Campbell, I know you have your foreman, John Herrick, over there observing you cattle daily. I presume you do keep heat records on individual cattle"

"I sure do. Do you want to see the records?"

"I sure do."

We went into the kitchen of the ranch house. Mary Campbell produced a couple of cups of hot coffee and Frank Campbell and I sat down to examine the records.

"Mr. Campbell, the records show that these cows are settling but that early embryonic death is occurring. Look. The normal cycle of a cow is about twenty-eight days. If the bull wasn't any good, the cows would be coming back in heat every twenty-eight days. Instead, they are returning to heat between thirty-five to sixty days. This means that the bull is fertile but the embryos aren't surviving."

"Well, Dr. Porter, what is the cause of the trouble? I never had anything like this happen before."

"Where did you get the bull and how long have you had him?"

"I borrowed the bull from the Westview Polled Hereford Ranch over at Sedalia, Missouri. I traded him a good cow for the service of the bull. I couldn't wait until Rex Domino 167 is shipped the last of the year."

"You mean you people are loaning bulls back and forth?"

"Of course. There are only a few good bulls around. We have to share them."

"You also share your problems."

"What do you mean?"

"If anyone of you has a venereal disease in your herd, you are going to share it with your colleagues. Sexual promiscuity in any species including man is accompanied by venereal diseases. The dairymen went to artificial insemination years ago, partly to avoid this problem."

"You mean Westview loaned me an infected bull. Why the S.O.B.!"

"Did you ask him about the bull or examine the breeding records of the cows the bull had been used on?"

"No, but Westview should have been honest enough to not loan an infected bull."

"Well, it could be that the cows in the herd were immune to the disease so he didn't realize he was shipping you a diseased bull. On the other hand, your cows were not immune so they aren't settling."

"Do you mean that my cattle will get an immunity?"

"Probably. You may well have vibriosis, which is carried by bulls on a permanent basis unless successfully treated but to which cows will develop an immunity if given breeding rest after exposure. You should always first use a new bull with an unknown breeding history on a few heifers that have never been exposed to a bull to determine if the bull is indeed free of any veneral disease. If the heifers settle, then you can be reasonably confident when you turn the bull loose with your other cows."

"Hell. Dad never had this trouble, and he dealt with cattle all his life. He was always trading bulls."

"Well, you've got the problem now."

"Dr. Porter, I've got to get these cows settled to get ready for the sale. If anything happens to upset that sale, it'll take me years to recover."

"Well, first, you've got to give these cows breeding rest so they'll clear up their infections. Second, you've got to use a bull you know is clean or else go to artificial insemination."

"What about Domino Star 23rd?"

"We can try treating him or you can take him back to Westview."

"Dr. Porter, what are you doing tomorrow?"

"Well, I had an appointment to do some work out at Boyd Wilson's, but I could get out of it or send my father over. Why?"

"Let's go to Centralia tomorrow. That's where Rex Domino 167 is. They do artificial insemination there. Maybe they'll have some frozen semen we can start using."

"O.K. What time do you want to start out?"

"I'll be by about 6:00. We can eat on the way. It's about a three-hour drive."

The next day we drove to the home of Rex Domino 167 who was to make history at Fredonia in ways that were not foreseen on that date. They did indeed have some frozen semen that we could have since Frank Campbell had already contracted to purchase the bull. The breeding association had restrictions on the use of frozen semen. One of the restrictions was tht semen could only be used by the owners of the bull on their own cattle, and another was that the semen could not be used after the bull died. Anyway, the frozen semen combined with several other measures did manage to solve the problem. The cows did get inseminated artificially or naturally. Plans went forward for the sale that was to make Frank Campbell's fame and fortune.

The sale was scheduled to follow the American Royal Livestock Show in Kansas City. It was one of four sales being held after this American Royal by Polled Hereford stockmen. The sales were on succeeding days, the premise being that the American Royal would attract enough buyers. It was further premised that these buyers would attend the four shows, since they would be held on succeeding days immediately after the Royal. The same auctioneer crew was to handle all four sales. The auctioneer and the four stockmen sent out joint advertising literature. Sales catalogues were prepared by each stockman and distributed to all interested and potential buyers. I worked with Frank Campbell getting the health papers ready. Finally nothing remained to be done but to wait for the appointed day.

The Campbell ranch was located the farthest from Kansas City. The Campbell sale was scheduled to be the fourth of the four sales.

The reports from the first three sales were that record crowds of buyers showed up and that record prices were paid for the stock. Frank Campbell was optimistically awaiting his day—the day he had been preparing for two years if not for his entire life. All Wilson County was looking forward to this spectacular show.

The day dawned bright and beautiful. During the night the auctioneer crew had moved in its show tent and bleachers from the premises where the sale had been held the previous day. At dawn's first light the tent crew started erecting the tent and setting up the bleachers. By 9:00 A.M. everything was in readiness and dozens of local stockmen and myself started gathering to witness how the big timers operated. All of us had attended many farm sales and many community barn sales, but none of us had ever witnessed a sale under a big top on a farm. It was just like attending a circus. This was going to be a great day for Wilson County and we wanted to be able to tell our grandchildren about it. The Ladies' Aid Society of the local Methodist church set up a stand to serve food and drinks.

The sale was to commence at 10:00 A.M. The local stockmen and I waited in anticipation of seeing what these millionaire stockmen looked like. We waited and we waited. A few showed up, but only a few. The start of the auction was deferred an extra hour but only a few more of the so-called big-time stockmen showed up and most of them came out of curiosity or courtesy, it turned out. At 11:00 A.M. the sale started and, because there was plenty of room on the bleachers, all the local stockmen got seats and prepared to watch the auction of these cattle that were to sell for thousands of dollars each.

The auction started. A few prime individuals were sold first to create the price climate for the ensuing sales. These individuals did fetch from $1,000 to $2,500 but not the $5,000 plus contemplated. The local stockmen began to nudge each other.

The auctioneer was cajoling the buyers. "What am I bid for this heifer? She's number 14 in your catalogue. Just look at that pedigree. She's got Royal Domino and Princess Ducaine blood flowing in her veins. Come on, what am I bid? Who'll make it $2,000? Two—two—two—who'll make it 2,000?"

The crowd sat on their hands. Nobody answered the auctioneer.

The auctioneer looked around at the stockmen who had attended the sales the previous three days. "Gentlemen, you were paying $4,000 and $5,000 for heifers like this yesterday over at Blue Valley and the day before at Pleasant Hill. This heifer is a bargain at $2,000. Who'll offer $2,000?"

Silence spread thoughout the tent.

"Gentlemen, gentlemen, look at the pedigree. This heifer could be the foundation animal in any herd in the country. Sparkman, you could use a heifer like this in your herd. What will you bid on her?"

"Five hundred dollars."

"Now Sparky, that's insulting to the Campbells and you know it. Make a reasonable bid."

"Five hundred dollars," he repeated.

"Sparky, we'll stay here all day before I sell these cattle for prices like that. Leaf through that catalogue. Look at the picture of Rex Domino on the front. Better yet, go back in the barn and look at Rex Domino himself. These cattle came out of Tom Campbell's herd. We've known Tom for years. These cattle have Domino and Royal Chesterfield blood scattered all through those pedigrees. Now what am I bid?"

"Six hundred dollars," Sam Barkley from over at Altoona raised his voice.

"Gentlemen, I'm asking $2,000."

"Six hundred dollars." Sam repeated his bid.

The local stockmen began to look at each other. Were they hearing right? Maybe, just maybe, they could buy some prime quality bloodlines at rock bottom prices. Where were the buyers that were going to be purchsing these cattle for $5,000 and $10,000 each? If those fifteen or twenty strangers on the front rows of bleachers were the bidders, they were strangely quiet.

"All right, I'll ask $1500. Who'll offer $1500? Come on Morton, she's a steal at $1500. Do I hear $1500?"

"Six fifty." Jim Harrison from south of town raised his voice.

The auctioneer spent the next ten minutes reviewing the pedigrees of the heifer and trying to coax a bid out of the big timers. His efforts were fruitless. He looked anxiously back at Frank Campbell who said nothing. Frank was probably too stunned to comprehend what was occurring. Seeing no succor from that quarter, he returned to soliciting bids and ended up selling the heifer for $750 to a John Parker, another Wilson countian.

The flood gates were down. The big timers sat on their hands and the locals started bidding on the cattle. Hour after hour the sale continued and the prices progressively got lower. Some heifers sold for as low as $240.

I have seen my plans turn out badly. I have seen other persons have unfortunate experiences. Such is life. However, I have never personally witnessed the collapse of the dreams of an individual in such a dramatic fashion as those of Frank Campbell that day.

A week later I was out at the ranch. Frank was in the hospital with hepatitis and Tom was running the place and trying to put the pieces back together.

"I told Frank not to schedule the sale at that time with three other sales ahead, but he wouldn't listen. The big breeders had already bought all they wanted by the time they got there. Frank didn't even line up somebody to start the bidding out. He was helpless when Sparkman and Bunker and those other so-called friends sat on their hands."

"They sure didn't sell well."

"I always had somebody to start the bidding on each animal at my sales. Frank didn't think it was ethical but, by God, it's not ethical to sell heifers for $240 that come out of Royal Chesterfield either. He would have been better off if he had bid them all back in through the bidder. At least then he would have had the cattle and would have only been out the cost of the auctioneer."

"I didn't know people had bidders helping them."

"Dr. Porter, in our business you have to. I used to use Walt Burnside from down near Waco and then when he had a sale I would return the favor. No sir, you don't make money on sales being ethical."

A couple of summers later I was called out to the north pasture by Frank Campbell. Rex Domino was dead. He had been killed in a fight with a neighbor's bull. The neighbor kept a long-horned bull in an adjoining pasture. The two bulls paced the intervening fence, pawing the ground and making dreadful bellowing noises at each other. Frank Campbell erected an electric wire fence on his side of the fence to keep the bulls apart. He asked the neighbor, Les Williams, to keep his bull in another pasture. Les figured his bull could take care of himself since he had a very respectable looking set of horns, so he did nothing. Finally the inevitable happened. Les's horned bull tore through the fence and took on Rex Domino. Rex Domino was a polled animal; that is, he had no horns. Further he was a show bull and still carried far too much weight. Rex Domino never had a chance. He died as a result of getting too hot, of stress, and of being bruised over most of his body.

I did the necessary examination and necropsy of the bull to fill out the insurance papers. Frank was not satisfied with obtaining this compensation. His dreams were completely shattered with the death of the bull that he expected to launch him to fame and fortune. He sued Les Williams for $17,500.

When the case came to trial, I had to testify as to the cause of death to the bull. I had never been in a courtroom before, so the experience was interesting for me. It was of further interest because I found a veterinary colleague in the courtroom that day who testified for the defense as to other possibilities that could have caused the death of the bull, such as poison weeds or blackleg. It was the only time that my testimony was ever weighed against that of another person in court. The jury found for the plaintiff, Frank Campbell, so they must have considered that my testimony carried greater weight than the smoke screen of other possible causes of death suggested by my colleague.

Furthermore, the defense challenged the valuation of the bull. They placed the tax appraiser on the stand. He testified that Frank Campbell had protested the $20,000 valuation suggested by the county appraiser for the tax rolls.

"But you advertise this bull as being worth $20,000."

"All registered cattlemen do that. Why, I would sell the bull to you today for $5,000. Want to buy him?"

The appraiser didn't have the available money to call his bluff so returned to the Court House for consultation. The bull's value went on the tax rolls at a lower price because of the county's policy in appraising registered stock. The court accepted the plaintiff's valuation of the bull nevertheless.

I regretted being put in the position of an expert witness in the case because I was a friend of the defendant. However, I had no other alternative. I left Fredonia to return to college at about this time.

Frank Campbell also left Fredonia shortly afterwards. Les Williams may have lost the case, but he stills resides in Fredonia. He probably had the last laugh when he saw Frank Campbell leave.

A Black Sheep

EVERY profession has its black sheep. The veterinary profession is no exception. Dr. Lester Mattinson was the black sheep of southeast Kansas. All practitioners have disgruntled clients that move on to other veterinarians. Most of us try to handle the situation as diplomatically as possible. Today, one may be seeing the animal of a former client of our colleague. Tomorrow, the situation may be reversed. Sometimes personality clashes occur between the veterinarian and the client. Often it is just a case of the animal not responding to the treatment regimen prescribed by the first veterinarian as fast as the owner would wish. However, in the case of black sheep like Dr. Mattinson, every disgruntled client that approached him presented an opportunity not only to gain a new client but to blacken the reputation of the former veterinarian. Presumably he believed that this would further enhance his own reputation and thus increase his business.

His basic approach to a new and disgruntled client was to assure the new client that the animal would certainly have died if the former treatment had been continued. Generally, he would embellish these charges with a new diagnosis in an attempt to point out the incompetence of the former veterinarian.

Dr. Mattinson managed a small animal hospital in Monroe. He erected an imposing hospital building on a main highway years before these structures became commonplace in rural areas. If a dog or cat didn't respond to the treatment of one of us country veterinarians or if we didn't find time to take care of it because we were out doctoring cows or pigs, the dog or cat might show up at Dr. Mattinson's. From there on things would happen.

"See this swelling on the jaw of Sampson. It's an abscess. I'm going to drain it and give it some antibiotic. You say Dr. Stevens saw him yesterday? Yes sir, that's what I would expect. It's lucky you came in here today or you would have had a dead cat. Yes sir, I don't see how some veterinarians can be so incompetent and continue in practice."

He was one of the first veterinarians in the area to get an X-ray machine, which is an extremely valuable piece of equipment. However, it could be valuable for ulterior purposes as well. In his case he did choose to use the X-ray machine for ulterior purposes. He collected a beautiful set of X-ray films showing fractures of the different bones. His prize was one showing a fracture of the right rear femur. When an appropriately sized dog limping on a rear leg was presented to him, he would take an X-ray and then would produce the film showing the fracture. Never mind whether it was a right or a left rear leg that the dog was limping on, the client couldn't tell an X-ray film of the right leg from the left.

"Yes sir, it's a bad fracture of the femur. Here, let me attach this picture to the viewing screen so you can see for yourself. See that fracture of Bruno's right femur just below the acetabulum?"

"Oh, that's horrible. No wonder he is limping. He must be suffering terribly."

"Oh, he is! He is! It is a good thing you brought him in now. Another day and gangrene would have developed. The leg would have had to have been amputated then."

"Oh, Dr. Mattinson, I don't want anything to happen to dear Bruno. What can we do?"

"Well, I have a special traction splint to use on these cases. You leave him with me for three weeks and he'll be as good as new."

"Anything for Bruno. Oh, thank you, thank you, Dr. Mattinson."

"That's what I'm here for. I'll need a fifty-dollar deposit now. The balance can be paid when Bruno is released."

"Certainly, Dr. Mattinson. How much will be the bill be?"

"One hundred fifty dollars, plus hospitalization of two dollars per day, plus any other costs that may arise from unexpected complications."

"Gee, Dr. Mattinson, Dr. Martin only charged seventy-five dollars to splint our little Mary's arm. Isn't that a little expensive?"

"Now, Mr. Brown, see where this fracture is? This is going to require the use of my special traction splint to correct. You wouldn't want Bruno to develop gangrene and have to have the leg amputated, now, would you?"

"Oh, no. No. Here's the deposit money. I can see Bruno every day, can't I?"

"Now, Mr. Brown, your visits would only upset Bruno. It would only delay healing with Bruno jumping around every time you visited. You wouldn't want that, now, would you?"

"Oh, no. Of course not, Dr. Mattinson. I can telephone every day about him, can't I?"

"You certainly can, Mr. Brown. I'll be happy to keep you informed on Bruno's progress."

Most of my knowledge of what occurred at Dr. Mattinson's hospital was obtained from clients who were unsatisified with my services and ended up at Dr. Mattinson's. If the pet lived, it was because they had taken it to Dr. Mattinson's. If it died, it was because the pet hadn't been taken to Dr. Mattinson's in the first place. There was no way my colleagues or I could win. Heads we lost. Tails Dr. Mattinson won.

The most enlightening information I ever received on what transpired at Dr. Mattinson's was from Jack Shipley. One day I was out at Jack's dairy removing a particularly "ripe" retained placenta from one of his Holstein cows.

"Doc, Spot's begining to smell a little strong. I'm not about to stick my arm in there, so I called you."

"Well, that's the right thing to do, Jack. I do have protective sleeves and gloves to wear."

"I expect I could buy those too, Doc. It's just that I wouldn't know what to do after I got my arm inside."

"Well, I have had a little training and experience, Jack."

"Bob Black, down the road, would have tied a brick to the placenta and let the weight of the brick do the work."

"Bob doesn't have a Grade A dairy and doesn't care how soon his cows get settled again."

"Well, Doc, that isn't the whole story. The truth is that Bob doesn't do the milking down there. His wife, Betty, does. If Bob had to smell those cows after his brickbat treatment, he might call you, too. As long as he can get Betty to do the milking without complaining, he isn't going to give you any business."

By this time I had my right arm up inside Spot's uterus attempting to "unbutton" the placenta from the cotyledons. Spot was objecting by humping and straining, trying to expel my arm from her insides.

"Jack, you're just using one hand to hold that tail. Take the other hand and squeeze down over her backbone to make her quit straining."

"O.K. Spot didn't strain that much when the inseminator was pipetting her. You don't have the touch, Doc."

"Maybe my arm is bigger than that pipette."

"I guess so. We sure took a lot of pleasure away from the cows when we got rid of the bulls and started using inseminators. Those plastic pipettes may get the sperm in there but they just can't feel like the real thing."

"You wouldn't want the bulls back, would you?"

"Hell, no!" He changed the subject. "Say, Doc, how come you didn't go to a bigger town and go into the dog and cat business like Doc Mattinson did?"

I looked up over the rear end of Spot from my crouched position at Jack. "Why do you think that Dr. Mattinson has it so good?"

Jack grinned. "Well, you sure wouldn't find him with his arm up the rear end of a cow. He might sell the owner a couple of pills to put inside the cow, but that would be it."

"How do you know so much about what he would do?" My curiosity was aroused.

Jack had to laugh. "I guess you don't know anything about my working for Doc Mattinson."

"No, I sure don't. When did this all happen?"

"I think you must have been away at college. I had just finished high school and went down to Monroe to work for Doc Mattinson."

"You did? He does have a nice place, doesn't he?"

"He does. It impressed me when I first entered his office."

"Well, tell me more. How does he do?"

"He's practically coining money down there. It's legal larceny. But, Doc, you could make money conducting a legitimate practice with the dogs and cats."

My ears were now straining to catch every word. "What do you mean, legal larceny?"

Jack was still grinning. "Doc, my hand is getting tired squeezing on Spot's back. I could probably tell stories of what happens down there that would keep you here until tomorrow listening. I'll talk if you don't prolong your job.

"I promise. Start talking."

"Well, you know that pet cemetery Doc Mattinson has?"

"I have heard about it, yes."

"He has a beautiful coffin that he buries the dogs in."

"Did you say coffin or coffins?"

"I said coffin." Jack was laughing. "He sells that coffin for one hundred dollars. You can count the number of graves in that cemetery and determine how many times that coffin has been sold."

"You know what you're talking about?"

"I ought to. I had to transfer the bodies from that coffin to a box each time."

"What if the family accompanied the body to the grave?"

"That was no problem. Doc just sent me back that night to open up the grave and retrieve the coffin. Hell, that coffin was custom made. He wasn't about to buy a new one each time."

"What about the tombstones?"

"Well, they couldn't be reused obviously once the words were chisled on them. However, I'm sure he made a nice markup on those, too."

"Maybe we ought to go into that business here in Fredonia. You got an acre out near the road we could hedge in and use."

"I could do that, but I don't want to be a part of selling the same coffin over and over again. Besides, I don't like to have to bury dogs twice."

"The problem is that I don't know very many people in Fredonia who would pay for the coffin the first time. I have enough trouble getting $7.50 for a spay operation. I guess I'm just not a good salesman."

"You could hospitalize dogs. Doc pays his overhead hospitalizing dogs that aren't sick."

"What was he getting for hospitalizing dogs?"

"I don't remember the exact figure, but he was charging twice as much for hospitalizing as for boarding dogs. He wasn't giving any special treatment to the hospitalized dogs. Since he wasn't losing any money for boarding dogs, he sure had to be making a nice profit on hospitalization. He advertised that the dogs were under care twenty-four hours a day. Since I had a room up above, I was supposed to be the night nurse. Hell, I practically never went back into the 'hospitalization ward' after I closed up for the day, but since I was staying above I guess you could say that the animals were under care—that is, under me. Funny, huh, Doc?"

"I guess I'm too honest, but I don't think Fredonia has enough potential clients to get by with that type of activity."

"Doc, you just need me as an office boy for a week and I'll educate you. By the way, my hand is getting tired. Aren't you about through?"

"Sure, I was just holding it inside to give you a chance to talk. Here it comes."

With that I removed my arm and dragged the separated placenta out in my clenched fist. After cleaning up and replacing my things in my car, I drove back to town. As I recalled the odor from the "ripe" retained placenta, I wondered if indeed I shouldn't have gone to a larger town and entered a legitimate small animal practice.

"Matilda's in Labor!"

MILK goat people are a different breed of humanity. Their sentimental attachment for goats is equivalent to that which persons have for their dogs and cats. Furthermore, the goats sense this love and respond in kind by following their owners around, licking their fingers, or demonstrating in other ways their affection. Dairymen often name their cows; however, they seldom become sentimentally attached to them. If a cow develops an incurable case of mastitis (infection of the mammary glands) or fails to settle, off she goes to the packinghouse. Goat owners would never consider such action. I often suspected that these men would divorce their wives before selling a goat, but this is not a fair assessment. They are, as I said earlier, a different breed of people and I love them for it. If I ever developed a specialty practice, and there were enough goat owners in the area to justify it, I would develop a goat practice.

The primary reason for the promotion of milk goats is because some people cannot tolerate cow's milk and others just prefer goat's milk to cow's milk. Moreover, most of these people do not want the milk pasteurized; they wish to drink it raw. This is fine except for two points. First, the milk must be from goats that are free from diseases communicable to man and must be handled with special precautions so that the bacteria are kept at an acceptable level. Because of the dangers that can accompany the consumption of raw milk, most municipalities require that milk be pasteurized before it is sold. This brings me to the second point—in most places it is illegal to sell milk that is not pasteurized. For people who desire raw milk and are not in a position to keep a goat on their premises, this presents a problem.

One of my clients attempted to handle this problem in a unique manner. He had been providing raw milk to some persons desirous of obtaining such a product. After discussions on the subject, we decided that it would be wise for him to TB and brucellosis test his goat herd to assure the consumers of the milk, including his family, that they would contract neither disease from the consumption of the milk. Accordingly, I tested the herd. The bloods were sent to the state laboratory for the conduction of the serologic test for brucellosis. The entire herd was negative for tuberculosis and brucellosis. This, I thought, was the end of it. However, I was mistaken. A few weeks later a state regulatory official showed up at my client's premises.

"Are you John Smith?"

"That's what I answer to. I see you're driving a state car."

"That's right. I work for the Department of Agriculture."

"Then I presume you aren't here on a social call."

"You could say that."

"Well, what have I done to attract the governor's attention?"

"I don't know that you have done anything wrong, and I hardly think the governor is aware or will be aware of this visit."

"Would you like a cup of coffee?"

"Well, I could drink some. It has been a few hours since breakfast."

"Fine. Come on in. Mildred always has a pot on the stove. We can talk at the kitchen table."

John opened the back door and directed the official into the kitchen.

"Mildred, this is Mr. . . . I'm sorry, I didn't get your name."

"I didn't give it to you. I'm Bob Sanders."

"Bob, this here is Mildred, the woman I've been married to for nigh onto twenty years. Right, Mildred?"

"I'm pleased to meet you, Mr. Sanders. I wish John wouldn't bandy that twenty years stuff around so much. It makes me feel old."

"You're like my wife. She says she is never going to get past thirty-nine. I don't know how we're going to handle it on our silver wedding anniversary though. She's going to have to acknowledge to being over thirty-nine or claim we were married when she was fourteen."

"Yes, we women do have problems, don't we. Please draw up a chair and sit down. You will have some coffee, won't you, Mr. Sanders? I know John wants some."

"Yes, I would. That coffee smells good and, as I was telling your husband, it has been a few hours since breakfast."

"How will you have your coffee, Mr. Sanders, black or white?"

"With lots of cream. I have to support the dairy industry here in the state."

"That's fine. You'll drink it with cream from goat's milk in this house."

"Fair enough."

Mildred set two cups on the table and poured the coffee from a pot that had been simmering on a back burner of the kitchen stove.

She then took a cream pitcher from the refrigerator and set it on the table next to a sugar bowl. The two men drew up chairs and proceeded to whiten their coffee. Mildred went back to her kitchen chores.

"Now, Bob, to what do I owe the honor of this visit?"

"Well, Mr. Smith, remember that blood test you had run on your herd last month?"

"Sure. My herd was clean, wasn't it?"

"Yes, it was. The reason I'm here is because you must be selling milk, and you aren't registered as a Grade A milk dealer."

"That's wrong and that's right."

"You said that was wrong and that was right. Would you care to elaborate?"

"Sure I will. It's simply because I do not sell milk so I'm not registered as a Grade A milk dealer."

"Now, Mr. Smith, you can't possibly drink all that milk here. What do you do with it?"

"I don't own those goats, Bob. I just board them and milk them for the owners. They come and pick up the milk."

Bob Sanders took a sip of coffee and pondered this information. "I presume you can show me some documentation to that effect."

"Certainly." John arose and left the room. In a few minutes he was back and threw a stack of papers on the table in front of Bob Sanders. "Here are the contracts with the owners all duly signed and notarized. Read them over. They are all legal."

Bob Sanders leafed through the documents. They confirmed what John had told him. He smiled and looked across at John now seated and finishing his coffee. "You've thought of everything, haven't you?"

"Well, I didn't want to break the law."

"You wouldn't mind showing me your milking parlor, would you?"

"Of course not. When you finish your coffee, we're off."

A short time later they were at the milking parlor. Bob Sanders had a quizzical look on his face.

"Mr. Smith, do you know what the requirements are for a Grade A milking parlor?"

"Can't say that I do, Bob. Would you like some pictures here as an example?"

"I'm afraid that any pictures I'd take here would have to be used as an example of what not to do."

"Now, Bob, look at these raised milking platforms. That showed a lot of ingenuity, didn't it?"

"Yes, but look at this dirt floor. That would never be acceptable in a Grade A dairy."

"Now, Bob, I don't milk on the floor. I milk into buckets."

"Mr. Smith, dirt floors just aren't conducive to producing milk with a low bacteria count."

"The owners of these goats aren't complaining. As far as I know, none of them are sick."

"Another thing, Mr. Smith, you should have a closed-in room adjoining this milking parlor with a cooler and place to wash and store your milking equipment."

"Bob, we do that all up at the house."

"Mr. Smith, you may be legal in your paperwork but your type of operation is slightly out of date."

"Bob, as long as the owners aren't complaining, I can't see as it is any concern of the state."

Bob Sanders had to smile. "You may be right, Mr. Smith, but I think you'd find a concrete floor and an adjoining cooling and clean-up room of great convenience to you."

"Well, Bob, I'll think about it."

"Mr. Smith, while you're thinking about it I'm going to have to visit with our legal counsel in relation to your activity. I'll get back in touch with you."

"Anytime, Bob. Always want to be legal."

After some further conversation regarding the weather and about the price of grain, Bob Sanders got into his car and drove off, leaving John chuckling to himself.

One evening I received a call from Ben Hodges just as I was finishing supper. "Doc, can you come out? Matilda is in labor and is having problems."

I knew without asking that he was talking about one of his milk goats. "Sure, I'll be there in a few minutes."

When I drove into the yard, Ben met me as I got out of the car. "Sure glad you could get here, Doc. Hazel says Matilda has been in labor since about 4:00 P.M. Ain't like Matilda to have problems. This is her fourth freshening and the only time she ever had trouble delivering."

"Ben, I guess we had better take a look. Where is Matilda, out at the barn?"

"Yep. Can I help you carry anything, Doc?"

"No, but you can get some warm water and soap and a towel."

"Hazel's got it ready. I sure hope Matilda gets along all right. She's our best milker."

When we arrived at the barn, I found Matilda loose in a box stall. Hazel joined us promptly. I stripped off my shirt and proceeded to wash my hands.

"Ben, tie Matilda up in the corner and hold on to her tail. I'll need to make an examination."

"Got you, Doc."

After cleaning up the rear of Matilda, I washed and lubricated my hands. Next I inserted a hand into the vagina to determine what the difficulty was. I felt a nose and a number of feet.

"Ben, we've got too many feet here."

"Now, Doc, Matilda always has twins. She should have eight feet in there."

"Maybe so, but they can't all come at once."

"Dr. Porter, you'd better get those feet straightened out," Hazel chimed in. "Ben will be mighty hard to live with if anything happens to Matilda."

"Doc, you know how it is. Matilda just has a sweeter disposition."

"Now, Ben, you're no angel yourself."

In the meantime, I was attempting to match up one or two of the feet with the nose protruding into the vagina. If a foot didn't seem to have a connection with the protruding nose, I'd push it back. Finally I ended up with two feet, a head, and ample working room. "O.K., Ben, let's get this kid out of here."

I started pulling on the feet. When they were extruding from the vagina, I instructed Ben to pull on the feet while I reinserted my hand to guide the head through. In a few moments a kid lay at our feet. I cleared the mucous from the nose and mouth and turned it over to Hazel to rub down and dry with some hay and burlap sacks.

"That ought to solve the problem, Ben. Let's give Matilda a few minutes rest. She ought to deliver the other one without problems."

"What you got there, Hazel, a boy or a girl?"

"Got a little boy, Ben. It looks just like Romeo."

"It should. Romeo is the daddy."

"Yes, sir, Ben. Every one of Romeo's babies have that black star on the forehead."

"Doc, it looks like Matilda is getting ready to deliver the next one."

"I wouldn't be so sure, Ben. That's a tail. She may need some help if some back feet aren't up there too."

I reinserted my hand. No feet were present—just a rear end and tail. As the pelvis seemed small, I pushed the rear end forward and worked my hand forward underneath the kid's body to grasp the feet and straighten them out into the pelvis. This done, Matilda cooperated by expelling another kid.

"Ready for another one, Hazel?" Ben was smiling. Matilda was going to be all right.

After cleaning up the mucous from the nose and mouth from the new arrival, I turned it over to Hazel. I then washed my hands and made a cursory examination of Matilda's vagina. Feeling nothing, I cleaned up and left, leaving Ben and Hazel with Matilda and the twins.

The next morning the telephone rang about 7:00 A.M. Marian was preparing breakfast. I answered.

"Doc, is that you?"

"Yes. How's Matilda doing, Ben?" I could always recognize his nasal twang.

"Oh, she's doing fine. Remember those twins Matilda delivered?"

"Sure, how are they doing?"

"Well, they're doing fine too, but they ain't twins, they're quadruplets."

"They're what?"

"They're quadruplets. Matilda had two more kids during the night." I could hear Ben laughing uproariously.

"Well, I'll be damned."

"That's what Hazel said too. She's having to bottle feed the two extra."

"I must have left too soon."

"No, Matilda didn't have any more trouble. You don't give rebates on things like this, do you?" Ben again laughed heartily.

"Well, I haven't gotten involved in rebates yet. You'll have to give Romeo a medal for distinguished service."

"Hazel doesn't think so. She thinks it's a nuisance to bottle feed the extra kids. She says I'm going to have to have a talk to Romeo about not getting over-involved in his romances in the future."

With that he hung up. I sat there shaking my head. How was I to know Matilda had two more kids. I couldn't get my hand past the vagina to any extent, and she certainly looked hollowed out on the side after the delivery of the twins.

An event occurred a few months later that proved far more embarrassing. I was called over to Altoona to examine a doe goat, Mabel, belonging to the Baptist preacher. She was due to kid and kept straining and passing water but nothing occurred. I made an examination, but the cervix was still closed. She had a full udder and seemed healthy so I thought it best not to hurry nature along. I advised Reverend Thomas Taylor to be patient and wait a day or two.

Two days later Reverend Taylor telephoned. "Dr. Porter?"

"Yes, this is Dr. Porter."

"This is Reverend Taylor. Remember Mabel?"

"I certainly do, Reverend Taylor. How is Mabel doing?"

"Just the same as when you were over here, Dr. Porter. She is still straining. What are we going to do?"

"Gee, I don't know." I really was puzzled. Mabel was apparently ready to kid but nothing was occurring. "Why don't you bring Mabel over to the office and I'll examine her again?"

"Sure, Dr. Porter. I certainly don't want anything to happen to her. I can't live without goat's milk."

A couple of hours later he showed up with Mabel riding proudly in the back seat of his sedan. Another examination revealed an apparently pregnant doe straining to deliver but with no dilation of the cervix. I discussed the situation with Reverend Taylor.

"Reverend Taylor, I frankly don't know what we have here. I'm afraid to let her go any longer. I'm going to suggest that I perform a caesarean."

"Dr. Porter, I'm really worried about Mabel. If you think that's the best thing to do, go ahead."

Mabel was taken to surgery and prepped. After strapping her to the table and giving a tranquilizer and local anesthesia, I made an incision in front of her udder into the abdominal cavity. Quickly, I reached inside to guide the pregnant uterus to the outside. All I felt were coils of intestines, eagerly trying to get past my hands and to the exterior. Horrors! Where was the uterus?

Further examination revealed a shrunken uterus curled up in front of the pelvic cavity. It still had some fluid in it but most had been passed during the straining of the past few days. No fetus was present in the uterus. The Reverend was certain that Mabel had not aborted or delivered a neonatal fetus. The closed cervix would indicate that his observations were right. The embarrassing diagnosis I had to make was that of a false pregnancy. It's very difficult to explain why a caesarean was performed on a nonpregnant doe—especially to a Baptist preacher.

Caught in the Rising Water

It was June 28, 1956. It was a beautiful Sunday afternoon. That morning my wife had given birth to our third child—our first and only son—without complications. The first child's birth had been a difficult presentation; the second had been a stillbirth. I was elated to become the father of a boy and to have Marian go through childbirth without complications. I could still remember standing beside Dr. Ralph Wilson at the time of the birth of the first child and offering suggestions as to how I would have handled the presentation. It was a breech presentation. I told Dr. Wilson that if I was handling the case I would have straightened the rear legs out to facilitate delivery. Dr. Wilson was noncomittal; somehow he didn't think my method of delivering breech presentations in calves was applicable to the case at hand, mainly Marian. The first born, a daughter, was delivered rear end first with her legs doubled up along her body. The only real advantage I could see to Dr. Wilson's method of handling the breech presentation was that the doctor could determine the sex of the offspring early in the delivery process. Anyway, everything had gone smoothly this morning. I was the father of a son to bear the Porter name.

That afternoon I was headed for Tex Larkin's ranch to look at a sick cow. Tex's ranch was located some twenty miles west of Fredonia. It would be a beautiful drive up through the timbered hills area. The pastures would be green with grass, the top of the hills would be covered with oak trees, the wild flowers would be in bloom along the roadside, cattle would be grazing in the pastures or lying along the fences—it promised to be a relaxing drive. Tex was a middle-aged, congenial rancher who ran a small spread with about a hundred head of cattle. He always had the animals to be examined confined in a corral upon my arrival. He expected me to stop and have a glass of iced tea and some small talk with him before leaving. When I told him I had become a father that day, I could expect that he would at least find a couple of cans of cold beer to toast the event. Maybe he would even find some bourbon. I expected no more calls for the day; if so, Armer would take them. I had promised Marian to come back to the hospital to see her that evening. Yes, it was a beautiful day.

I drove west out of Fredonia. Four miles along the road I had the choice of taking the regular route or a shortcut. The shortcut would save only about two miles and it ran over a low-water bridge, but it was a scenic crossing of the river. The river had been at low water for several weeks and there had been no recent rains so I anticipated no problem in making the crossing. Besides, the U.S. Corps of Engineers who regulated the water level at the Fall River Dam some twenty-five miles upstream would not be releasing any additional water into the river since no further rains were expected. I decided to indulge myself that day and take the shorter and more scenic route.

A mile further down the road I slowed down when I approached the river bank overlooking the low-water bridge. There was indeed water running over the bridge floor, but the concrete banisters on each side indicated that it was only a few inches deep. I drove slowly down the bank of the river onto the bridge. I had driven through water this deep on many occasions both in Kansas and in Mexico without incident. The secret was to drive slowly so as not to splash water up on the motor and drown it out.

I drove slowly out on the bridge. Everything seemed to be going as planned. I anticipated no trouble or I wouldn't have started across. Suddenly, when half-way across, the car motor spluttered and died. Consternation struck me. Here I was on a back road with a car drowned out on the middle of a water-covered bridge. How long would it be before someone might come along to offer me help. Should I wait or should I walk out to the nearest farm house and find assistance?

As I was pondering my decision, the water began rising over the floor boards of my car. This was a revolting development. The Corps of Engineers must have been releasing water from the Fall River Dam and I was caught in a surge of water from that release. Persons using the bridge crossed at their own risk. I risked the crossing and now I was caught. Furthermore, I didn't know how high the water might rise. Should I wait it out or should I wade and then walk out for assistance? The water rising over the floor boards dictated that I had to move from my present position, regardless. I climbed through the car window and up on to the roof top to ponder the situation and my decision.

It had been my own recklessness that led to my present predicament. I could blame no other person. I recalled the time I was driving north out of Fredonia and had to cross the Verdigris River to make a call. The Verdigris was out of its banks. I had to make a decision as to where it would be possible to cross. I drove straight north towards the river. As I passed Bill Harlin's farm, I could see the water across the road up ahead. Bill and some of his neighbors were standing by the roadside so I pulled over and stopped.

"Bill, I've got to get across the river. Can I get through here?"

"Ha! Ha!" Bill was always laughing. "Sure you can go through."

I was in a hurry so I started up and drove north into the water. A few hundred feet further the water drowned out my motor and I found myself stalled. Bill went back up to his farmyard, started his tractor, and drove up to pull me back out of the high water.

"Bill, why in the living hell did you tell me I could get through?"

"Why, Doc, I didn't think anybody in their right mind would try to drive through. I thought you knew I was kidding."

"Damn, Bill, when I ask you information, I want a straight answer. If I had known, I wouldn't have asked you."

"Don't get mad, Doc. There won't be anybody crossing the Verdigris north on this road for four or five days—and that is if it doesn't rain again."

Anyway, I could blame Bill Harlin for that misadventure. This time I could blame nobody but myself. I sat there and debated with myself about what to do. The afternoon that had started out so beautifully quickly began to lose its charm. The river current seemed to be running rather rapidly, so I sat and waited rather than trying to wade out for help. Thirty, maybe forty-five minutes later a pickup with a couple of young farm couples pulled up to the bridge. They recognized me and saw my plight.

"Dr. Porter, we don't have a tow chain along. You wait and we'll go down to Charley Moyer's and get a chain."

I readily agreed. I hardly had an alternative but to wait, but it was polite of them to word the order as if I did.

Later they returned with the tow chain to hook on my rear bumper. First they knotted a throw line onto the tow chain. Next they threw the line to me, sitting on top of my car. I caught the line and slipped down into the water, holding on to my car through the opened windows and then, when I reached the rear, by the rear bumper. I pulled in the line and behind it the tow chain. When I had pulled enough of the tow chain across, I tied it to the bumper supports and climbed back into the driver's seat of my car as my rescuers pulled me back out of the water.

Some dry rags were used to dry off the spark plugs and distributor points. Thirty minutes later I coaxed the motor into sputtering and then into coughing and starting off. After thanking the young couples for coming to my assistance, I retraced my route and started back up through the timbered hills on the conventional route. It was now late afternoon but I had told Tex I would be there so I would go ahead.

When I arrived at Tex's ranch, I coud find nobody. I honked the horn of my car, I looked around the corrals and the stables, but no Tex and no sick animal. I sat and waited for an hour. Probably Tex had gone over to a neighbor's and would return shortly since I told him I would be there that afternoon. An hour passed and still no Tex. It was now getting to be early evening. The day was getting to be more unpleasant as time passed. I was suppposed to see Marian that evening, and here I was sitting out at a deserted ranch with the night fast approaching. Disgustedly, I started the car and drove back to Fredonia.

I arrived in Fredonia too late to go see Marian. When I stopped by the hospital the next day, an unhappy Marian greeted me.

"Why weren't you here yesterday evening when I needed you so much? I was really feeling low and you were out having fun with the boys."

"Marian, I was sitting on top of a drowned out car on the low-water bridge and then in a deserted farmyard all afternoon."

"A likely story. You were probably down at Harry's drinking beer while I wasn't feeling well."

"Now, Marian."

"You men are all alike. We women deliver the children and suffer and you celebrate."

"But, Marian . . ."

Two weeks later I showed Marian a snapshot I received in an envelope in the mail. It showed me sitting on the top of a car at the low-water bridge with water swirling around the car.

"Marian, here's something I received in the mail this morning. It shows where I was the afternoon of Craig's birth."

"Oh, Jim, is that you?"

"Of course it's me. That's what I was trying to tell you."

"Well, I never know when to believe you. Just be sure you have snapshots to back you up when you tell stories like that one."

"Yes, Marian."

Sadie, the Snake Lady

DOCTOR, look what's coming this way!" Clarence and I were loading my station wagon preparatory to leaving for the country on our morning calls. I was at the back of the office loading vaccine and ice cubes into our picnic icebox. Clarence was just going out the door when he hollered at me.

I walked to the front of the office and looked out the window. A carnival had moved onto the fairgrounds the previous night. Approaching my office was a bathrobe-clothed woman with a large snake draped around her neck. She addressed Clarence, who was standing slightly aghast, as she neared.

"Is this a veterinarian office?"

"It sure is," Clarence answered.

"Are you the vet?"

"No. He's inside." Clarence opened the door for her and her snake and followed her inside. He was open mouthed, looking at the spectacle immediately in front of him. The woman, in her forties, wore a faded red bathrobe and probably not too much underneath. She had a round weather-beaten face that obviously had seen better days and probably needed a considerable amount of makeup to make her attractive. She had not yet applied her paint. Long red hair draped down her back. She wore a pair of thongs to protect her feet. A snake, possibly four or five feet long, was looped around the back of her neck and hung down over the front of each shoulder. The snake lazily raised its head and protruded its tongue in Clarence's direction as it passed.

"Good morning, you a vet?" she asked.

"Yes, I'm Dr. Porter. How can I help you?" Like Clarence, I could feel my mouth gaping open.

"I'm Sadie Milton and this boa here is Lucifer. Say hello to Dr. Porter, Lucifer."

Lucifer flicked out his tongue at me and then dropped his head on Sadie's ample right breast. Lucifer's tail was draped over the left breast. Sadie was fully endowed in that department and the snake's head and tail amplified that endowment. I was not used to having women clothed only in bathrobes enter my place. The presence of Lucifer made it even more of an unusual event.

"Hello, Lucifer. Now what can I do for you? It isn't often I'm honored by a visit from a lady wearing a snake."

"You'll excuse me for not having my war paint on, but we had a long night moving over from Joplin. I just got up and I was so worried about Lucifer. He hasn't eaten in several weeks. I've tried chicken, rats, birds, anything I can think of. He acts hungry but he just won't eat. I saw your shingle hanging out in front this morning so came over."

"If you had waited another ten minutes, we'd have been gone. Bring Lucifer on back to the table."

"You've got a nice place here, Doc. Treat many snakes?"

"Can't say that I do. They kill snakes around here."

"I won't let them kill Lucifer. Picked up Lucifer when I used to work for Maxy's Circus. He's really a dear. Go ahead and pet Lucifer's head. He likes that!"

She bent over the table, the better to place Lucifer's head near me. I reached over and gingerly patted his head. Lucifer, responding to my warm hand, raised his head. This released the pressure on the robe concealing the underlying breast. The robe fell open and a large pendulous breast was exposed. Clarence and I both unconsciously gasped.

Sadie remained nonplussed. "You fellows are gettin a bonus. Most men have to pay to get in my show over there on the Midway." She straightened up and nonchalantly pulled her robe back over the nipple of her breast and placed Lucifer's head back on top to serve as a clasp.

Regaining my composure, I asked, "You say Lucifer won't eat? How long has it been since he's eaten?"

"All of a month, Doc. I've tried everything. Sure hope you can do something. Most vets won't even look at a snake."

"I expect that's right. But I'm game. Can you handle his head so we can look at his mouth?"

"Whatever you say, Doc." She reached down for Lucifer's head and raised it up directly in front of me. Again the robe draped open, exposing the well-endowed breast and nipple. Lucifer's head was directly in front of my face, the exposed breast a few inches below. Clarence blushed and modestly turned his head.

"Will Lucifer bite?" I was worried by two things. First, would somebody walk in the door and catch me in this compromising position? Second, would Lucifer bite? He did have some long fangs.

"No, he won't bite." Sadie placed her hands on the upper and lower jaw easily exposing his cavernous mouth. A quick glance revealed a string running from the left fang back and into the esophagus.

"Let me examine his body." Sadie undraped Lucifer from around her neck and laid him on the table. With the removal of the snake, the only thing holding her robe together was the waist band. The robe flopped open and both breasts protruded. Lucifer lay on the table with Sadie, breasts exposed, holding him extended.

I gulped, gingerly reached under the breasts and palpated the snake's body working backward from the head. About one-third of the way back along the length of the body I felt the hard hump I was feeling for.

"Miss Milton, you hold Lucifer. I think we can help him."

"Anything you say, Doc." She threw her head around to get her hair out of the way and in so doing shook her breasts. "Don't let that bother you, Doc. Come over and see my show tonight, and I'll really show you a thing or two."

I grunted as I reached for a set of forceps. Adroitly grasping the string I saw fastened around the fang, I slipped the noose holding the string free from the fang and started pulling on the string. Grudgingly but slowly it began yielding to my tugging. With one hand I grasped the hard lump further down the body and tried to massage and work the lump forward. A few minutes later, I pulled a yo-yo, string attached, out of the snake's mouth.

"I'll be a son of a gun, Doc, you're good. If you ever need a recommendation for snakes, just say that Sadie Milton with the American Midway Shows gives you a gold star."

"Thanks. Not certain that I'll ever need it."

Sadie gathered Lucifer up, pulled her robe back together and started for the door. "Sam, the boss will be over to pay you. I'll have him bring you boys a couple of tickets for my show. Actually you've seen more here than I can show over there. The sheriff makes me wear pasties. However, Lucifer and I do some movements never before seen by human eyes. I didn't give you the movements today. Leave the wives at home and come out and see the real thing tonight." With that she went out the door leaving Clarence and me sheepishly grinning at each other.

The Skunk De-scenter Specialist

SOME of my farm clients possessed exotic pets. Raccoons and skunks were the most popular, although bobcats, foxes, and opossums were occasionally seen. Coyotes were plentiful in the area but were thought to kill livestock so they were not kept as pets. They were the object of organized and unorganized hunting. Many farmers carried rifles in a rack above and behind the seat in the cab of their pickup trucks so they could shoot coyotes when spotted. The carcasses of coyotes could be seen suspended from fenceposts as one drove down the country roads, attesting to the success of the hunters. The successful hunters could be identified by reading the local newspaper to see who collected bounty at the county courthouse for how many pairs of coyote ears.

Opossums never become friendly so were generally kept for only a short time—as novelties—while they had young clinging to the nipples within their marsupial pouch. The young of opossum, as other marsupials, are born premature and must spend an additional period after leaving the uterus in the marsupial pouch before being ready to face the external world.

I was occasionally called on to spay or castrate some of these unusual pets. Some of the species, like cats, have unusual sensitiveness. Cats are especially susceptible to products containing phenol. I found to my consternation that bobcats are sensitive to lindane, a fly repellent. After castrating one young bobcat, I applied a product containing lindane to the wound as a screwworm repellent. The bobcat had been anesthetized with ether. It became conscious practically immediately and nearly tore my place apart with convulsive seizures. I avoided lindane like the plague after that.

The exotic species I worked on more than all the others was the skunk. Litters of skunks were often dug out of holes in the ground as a part of skunk-trapping activities.

Skunks are cute as kittens but if they are to be kept as pets, they had to be de-scented. No adult skunk, no matter how young it was when captured, is to be trusted with scent glands. Some persons ignored this advice but sooner or later an event occurred that made them regret this decision.

Most farmers in the area brought the young kittens to me to de-scent. Thus I became experienced though not sometimes as adept at the surgery as I would wish. Farmers could learn to castrate and dehorn their livestock. De-scenting skunks was not within their competency.

"Marian, look at this box I had Ike Smith make me." I showed her a wooden box, twelve by twelve by eighteen inches, with a glass window in the end that was hinged to the box and served as a lid.

"What in the world is that glass for?" she asked.

"Oh, that's to see whether or not the skunks are asleep."

"Skunks! I'd think you get enough of that. You always come home smelling after working on them."

"How do you know? Ceres doesn't tell you when I work on skunks. The only time you know is when I have an accident. Most times I don't have trouble, and you never know because I don't tell you."

"I know."

"Well, besides, I get good money for working on the skunks. I get five dollars a skunk. That's practically one dollar a minute and a lot of money."

"If it's so much money why do the other veterinarians send their clients clear over to Fredonia for you to work on?"

"They just don't know how to do it. I'm a specialist!"

"I think you ought to specialize in something else."

"Just wait. See this box? This is for anesthetizing skunks. I put the skunks and some cotton soaked in ether in this box and I can see when they're asleep."

"You still have to take them out of that box and take those scent glands out," Marian said dubiously.

"I'm way ahead of you. Clarence scavenged a window out of that house they were wrecking across the road. He put legs on it so we can now sit across from each other with Clarence holding the skunk under the glass while I reach under and do the surgery with the glass to protect me from any accident."

"I'll believe it when you come home without smelling horrible."

This conversation occurred one morning as I left for work. I had a chance to try out my equipment sooner than expected. That afternoon Clarence and I returned early from the calls.

Ceres smiled at me as I entered. "Doctor, I've got another surprise for you."

"What now?" I inquired somewhat hesitatingly.

"Well, Ken Larkins came by. He had this litter of skunks in a box. They are really cute. He left them here for you to de-scent. Said he was going up to the machine shop to have welded a piece that broke on his tractor. Said if you didn't have time, he would pick them up as he went home and bring them back another day."

"Yes, I expect when they're six months old and really smelly. How old are they?"

"They're just opening their eyes. What's that, about seven days?"

"I don't really know, but at least they're small. Clarence, let's get it done before we close up."

Sometime later I was proudly testing out my new equipment; the anesthetic box and the windowpane were to serve as a shield from the pungent spray. We were working in our large animal surgery room attached to the main office. Both of us were wearing plastic gloves. Clarence was presenting the rear end of the skunks to me with the tail held out of the way. I was deftly peeling the glands out by blunt dissection. I had progressed to the last skunk. No accidents had occurred. However, it just wasn't my day. On the last skunk I inadvertently cut the wall of the gland releasing the odiferous material. The windowpane did catch the spray but the odor was pungent enough to immediately permeate the room and our clothing. I finished the operation as quickly as possible before saying anything.

"Clarence, I guess I messed up on that last one."

"I guess you did. Well, that means Frieda will make me change clothes and take a bath before supper."

"I hope that's all Marian does to me. She is getting real testy about this skunk business I'm developing."

"Well, I think she should," said Ceres, who just then appeared at the door.

Later, when I arrived home, I was met by Marian at the door. She had a nose that could smell skunk odors a block away.

"Jim, you've been at it again. How could you tonight? You know we're supposed to go over to Chanute and see Eiliene and Cecil Cage installed as Worthy Matron and Patron of their Eastern Star chapter." Eiliene was my cousin who had refused to help me get a marriage license in Kansas City years before and Cecil her husband.

"It was only the last one I had trouble with."

"I don't care how many you had trouble with. You smell awful. They won't let you in the chapter room at Chanute. You will just embarrass me."

"Well, I won't go then. You go on over with the Jenkins."

"I guess I'll have to. You can baby-sit tonight instead of Sybil. Maybe you can get some of that odor scrubbed off before I get home tonight. There's a can of tomato juice in the ice box. If it's a miracle deodorant, here's a good chance to test it out."

"Now, Marian."

"Your supper is on the table. I'm staying away from you so I won't smell bad over at Chanute."

"Now, Marian, you won't smell."

"And furthermore, if you don't get that odor off, I'm sleeping on the couch downstairs when I get home tonight."

"Yes, Marian." I walked back into the kitchen to eat supper by myself and reflect on the trials attached to making a dollar a minute.

The Gentle Farmers

SALLY and Fred Smith retired from government service to farm. They had worked in Wichita for twenty-five years, Fred for the U.S. Postal Service and Sally for one of those three-letter agencies. Both were born on farms and they had always longed to return to a farm. Finally their dream was realized. They had saved their money and purchased eighty acres out southeast of Fredonia. They had enough acreage to pasture their few head of livestock and to raise some forage and grain for feeding. They built a small cottage that they kept well painted with constrasting colors for the window and door trims and immaculately clean inside. Sally had flower beds all around the house with beautiful flowers blooming at the appropriate times of the year. Fred, for his part, prided himself on the vegetable garden he planted and maintained. As he said, it provided them with most of the food they needed. The egg and milk money paid for the rest. Taxes weren't nearly as high as Wichita, and they did have their pensions.

When they first moved in about three years before, they had purchased a few chickens, sheep, and two milk cows. The milk cows were polled shorthorns. Neither Sally nor Fred liked to see anything hurt, so they decided to handle polled stock to eliminate the necessity of dehorning with its accompanying pain for the calves. I clamped their bull calves, eliminating the pain of castration with a knife. I also clamped their male lambs. The one thing I didn't do was dock the tails on the lambs. They just didn't want the lambs to undergo the pain of having their tails cut off. In those days I didn't have the foresight to realize that I could have done the operation under an epidural or even general anesthetic. Others farmers wouldn't have thought of using any method to eliminate the pain, however brief, and that was the environment in which I worked.

One warm August day I received a telephone call from Sally. "Dr. Porter, can you come quick? One of our lambs is eaten up with worms."

"Sure, I'll be right out." It had been a slow day and I was glad to get out of the office. Clarence climbed into the other side of the front seat of the station wagon and we were off to see the worm-eaten lamb.

A short time later Clarence was restraining the lamb while I examined the problem. Worms were indeed eating up the rear end of the lamb. Because it wasn't docked, the wool around the rear end of the lamb had become filthy and damp from contamination from fecal material and urine. The tail hung down over the area preventing air from drying the filthy mess. Infection and necrosis resulted, and flies had blown the area with their eggs. The eggs had hatched out into maggots (larvae), and these maggots were avidly eating all the dead flesh out. Actually maggot infection is not always such a bad thing because they eat only the dead tissue, thus cleaning up the area so natural healing can begin. Screwworms were a different thing. They invaded living tissue such as wounds and kept eating until they completed their larval development and dropped to the ground. Repeated blowing by screwworm flies could result in an animal literally being eaten alive. Fortunately the U.S. Department of Agriculture conducted a successful screwworm eradication program in this country and that fly is no longer a problem.

"You do have a bad situation here," I told Sally and Fred who were leaning over my shoulder to observe the gruesome area. "This is the result of not docking your lambs."

"I know. I know. We're just going to have to do it after this, Sally," Fred told her. "There isn't any way to do it painlessly, is there, Dr. Porter?"

"I could use an epidural but the pain from the epidural needle would probably be as much as that from the docking instrument. I use this instrument and the operation is over immediately. It separates the tissues and clamps the blood vessels at the same time so they won't bleed."

I clipped the area, removed the maggots with ether and forceps, and docked the tail so the area wouldn't get reblown by maggot flies. After we had finished, Fred invited me back to the cow barn.

"I want you to see our two cows, Betty and Caroline," Fred said. Betty and Caroline were standing in the shade back behind the barn lazily switching their tails. "Aren't they beautiful?"

They were indeed beautiful for show animals except they were milking cows. They weren't show animals. They must have weighed a ton, a full six hundred or more pounds above a normal weight for an animal in milk production. "They are beautiful, Fred, but at what fair are you planning to show them?"

"Oh, we don't show animals. Why do you ask?"

"They're way too fat for productive animals. You should put them on a diet."

"But they are always hungry and Sally and I don't like to see anything hungry."

"You and Sally aren't fat. In fact, you're real thin. If you can keep your food intake down, why don't you do the same for Betty and Caroline?"

"Oh, we're just not hungry. We eat all we want. But Betty and Caroline are hungry."

"I think Betty and Caroline have got you fooled. They know you'll feed them so they put on the hunger act. Besides, I expect they would give far more milk and be far quicker about settling if they got that excess weight off."

"The inseminator does complain about the weight on these cows," admitted Fred. "He says he has to make twice as many repeat trips on fat cows to get them settled. I know it does generally take about four heat periods to get them settled. The inseminator says it shouldn't take over one or two periods."

"He's telling you right," I said. "Sally seemed to be a little sad today. Anything wrong?"

"Why yes there is. I didn't know you'd notice it. Sally is about broken up. Patricia, our pet cat who was sixteen years old last January second, has disappeared. We've had her since she was just a small kitten. It is just like losing a member of the family. We haven't seen Patricia for a week. I suppose we'll get over it, but it is difficult."

"You get Sally another kitten," I advised. "That's the best cure."

"I suppose you're right, Dr. Porter," Fred agreed. "But if Sally should die, it'd be the same thing. I'd probably grieve myself to death. I couldn't go looking for another wife."

By that time we had returned to the car. "I'll be in Saturday and pay you, Dr. Porter."

I waved to Fred and to Sally who had rejoined him and drove back to the road and headed for town.

Sally and Fred did come in Saturday and caught me at my office. "Dr. Porter, I want you to take a look at a couple of my hens. They seem to be drunk."

"Bring them in and put them back on the table," I replied. "I'll be glad to take a look at them."

A few minutes later I was examining a couple of chickens that indeed seemed to be drunk. They were staggering, their wings were dropping, and their necks had completely lost the ability to hold their heads up. I'd lift up their heads by their neck feathers and let go. The heads would drop and I'd find myself with a handful of feathers.

"Those necks are sure limber, aren't they, Dr. Porter?" Fred said. "Suppose they got poisoned? Maybe the last batch of feed I got from the store was bad."

"I don't think so. Your chickens have limber neck."

"Limber neck? What's that?"

"They've been eating on something rotten and picked up a big dose of botulism poisoning."

"We don't have anything rotten around our place." Sally reminded me. "I couldn't stand the smell of anything dead."

"You must have something dead around there," I said. "Go down to the creek and look around. It may just be dead vegetation but you have to have something dead around. You're going to have more death losses until you remove the source of the trouble."

"Can you do anything for these two sick hens, Dr. Porter?" asked Fred. "I certainly don't like to see them die. Seeing something sick just breaks our hearts."

"There really is no treatment. I don't have much hope for the two hens but if they haven't eaten too much of the toxic material, they could live."

Sally retrieved the two hens and took them back to their car while Fred was paying the bill. "Never found Patricia?" I asked as Fred was leaving.

"No, sure didn't," Fred responded.

"You should get another kitten. It'll make you and Sally feel better again."

"You're probably right," Fred said as he walked out the door.

A few days later Clarence and I were passing the farm so I stopped. Sally walked out to meet me. "Dr. Porter, I've got something to show you."

I followed her back to a place south of their vegetable garden. "We found out what happened to Patricia. She died and we buried her here." She pointed to a small mound of dirt with a plank driven into the ground at the head of the grave. The plank had the name "Patricia" neatly lettered on it.

"You say Patricia died? But how?" I asked.

"It was what you said about the chickens. I don't know what

caused the death, but Fred got to looking and found Patricia's body down in the edge of the creek about two hundred yards south of the cow barn. She was pretty decayed and the hens were eating her up. It was horrible. Anyway we buried the last of her remains here, and the hens have stopped dying just as you said."

"It is sad, isn't it?" I agreed.

Sally was really feeling despondent. "Dr. Porter, I just couldn't send our beautiful cows, Betty or Caroline, to market. I'm going to let them die of old age here on the farm. We're all part of the family. Don't you think it would be nice to bury them here? I couldn't stand to have the dead animal truck pick them up."

Believing that the circumstances called for it, I agreed that would be the proper gesture.

As we were driving down the road, I remarked to Clarence on the sentimentality of Sally's attachment to their animals.

"That may be all right in its place," replied Clarence. "But I sure wouldn't want to be Fred and have to dig the hole to bury them in. That's going to be some hole."

"I'm Naming the Biggest after You"

COON Maxwell was a hound dog man. He had gone by the name Coon ever since I knew him. Coon, in this case, stood for raccoon just as possum stood for opossum. No self-respecting hunting man would call them anything but coons and possums. Coon's legal name was Mortimer. His parents took the name of some long deceased uncle to use in christening him. Coon never liked the name and never permitted any of his friends to call him that. When he was small they called him Mort. Later, when he reached his teens and had become an avid coon hunter, everybody got to calling him Coon. He took pride in that name as it related to his avocation and insisted that everybody call him Coon when he reached adulthood.

"Junior, can I bring Bear in?" It was Coon calling. I was just finishing my second cup of coffee as I didn't have anything pushing this morning. It was a cold and snowy day outside, so I wasn't likely to be too busy.

"Sure. Who's calling?" I asked. The voice sounded familiar but I couldn't place Bear.

"This is Coon Maxwell. Thought everybody knew my voice. Say, Bear, my blue tick coon hound, got his ear chewed up good by a coon he tangled with last night. It has been bleeding ever since. I think you had better look at it before you get started on your calls."

I agreed to meet him at the office in about twenty minutes. He lived about five miles out from town. He arrived driving his Ford pickup at the same time I was unlocking the front door. Bear was calmly sitting in the bed of the pickup, a bloody towel wrapped snugly about his head.

"Bear's a mess. Do you want to look at him in the truck or do you want me to bring him on in? He's going to get your floor bloody. He's bleeding like a stuck hog."

He did seem to be constantly dripping from the underneath part of the towel, but I told Coon to bring him on in. Clarence arrived and he and Coon brought Bear into the office and back to the examination table. Between the two of them they managed to hoist Bear up on the table without getting their clothes blood smeared.

"Let's take the towel off and take a look," I said.

"O.K., but it's really spurting. You'd better get ready to dodge the blood."

"All right. We can't do anything with it covered up."

Coon removed the towel and one small arteriole was still spouting blood a quarter inch or so each time the heart beat. Two or three others were oozing a little blood. The ear itself was split the entire length into two sections.

"Bear missed the neck when he grabbed for the coon. The coon got his ear and split it wide open." Coon was explaining what happened. "Bear sure never missed on that second grab. He was mad and finished that coon right off. Didn't get to see much of a fight and now this bloody ear to take care of."

"Do we need to put him out or will he hold still under a local?" I asked Coon.

"Junior, he'll never move, but give him a local anyway," said Coon.

After needling Bear with a local anesthetic, I clamped and ligated the spurter and cauterized the other oozers. I bandaged the ear tight against the head and told Coon to return the next week. Bear made an uneventful recovery albeit having a split ear. He still had some learning to do in regard to coon fighting or else he had the unfortunate luck of always treeing the meanest and biggest of the old boar coons.

A few weeks later Coon telephoned in the middle of the night. Marian shook me awake. "Jim, get that telephone or it's going to wake the baby. I was hours getting Darcy to sleep."

"Junior, it's me, Coon. Bear has done it again."

"What's he done this time?" I was trying to wake up and get my mind functioning.

"Tangled with another boar coon, he did. This time he got his leg all chewed up and I think it's broken. It swings from one side to the other when he moves."

"It's broken all right. I'll meet you at the office. Bring him on in."

"What is it this time?" Marian inquired. She was now wide awake.

"Coon Maxwell's dog, Bear, has got chewed up again. Coon likes to work all day and hunt all night. Doesn't seem to need any sleep. If this keeps up I'm going to have to recommend those veterinarians over at Chanute to him. I'll tell him they have excellent night facilities with a twenty-four hour attendant on duty. That ought to attract Coon."

"I wouldn't be so sure," Marian replied.

Some twenty minutes later I met Coon at the office.

"I am sorry to bother you, Junior, but didn't think I should let Bear go till morning. He's a damn good hunting dog, even if he does miss on that throat grab once in awhile."

With Coon restraining Bear I managed to anesthetize him with pentobarbital intravenously. While Bear was sleeping, I got the area cleaned, the fracture realigned using palpation (I had no X-ray), a Thomas splint fitted to the leg, and the area dressed and bandaged.

While I was thus involved, Coon kept up a constant monologue about his hunting activities. His hunt had been interrupted for the evening, but it was still early for him and he was exhilarated with the events of the evening prior to Bear getting his leg chewed up.

"You ought to come along with us sometime," said Coon. "Your Uncle Al is a great hunter and he has some mighty fine dogs. I think Bear has got some of Al Porter's dogs' blood in his veins."

"Al does like to hunt," I agreed. "When I first came back to Fredonia I took my wife hunting with him a couple of nights so she could have the experience. I think she enjoyed it, but the babies coming along have kind of cramped her activities in that field. You can't rock babies to sleep chasing after the coons."

"That's right," Coon agreed. "I went through the same experience myself. When my boys got big enough, they all enjoyed going with me. But now they've all left for the big cities and I'm back by myself again. My wife, Jennie, just isn't up to climbing up and down the hills anymore, let alone crossing creeks on fallen down trees. Junior, you'll have to join us some night for a hunt. Jack Parker, my neighbor over in the next section, and I go out regularly, weather permitting—and I guess sometimes when the weather isn't permitting. The dogs do have to be kept in shape, though."

"I'll take a rain check on that hunting. Got a 'gimpy' knee but remind me in a month. Might like to go. Speaking of keeping dogs in shape though, you must keep Bear tied up. He can hobble around on this crutch I splinted on him, but it's going to be awhile before he can chase coons again."

"How long do you think it'll be, Junior? Our other dogs are all right at trailing, but Bear is the best fighter. He gets chewed up once in awhile, but he's got courage. The other dogs are a little yellow. A big boar like the one that Bear will tackle will scare them away. We have to end up shooting the coon when Bear isn't there. That takes away a lot of the excitement."

"If you like that kind of excitement, you ought to go to the cock fights down in the barn near Independence," I said.

"I know. Sam Perkins raises those fighting roosters and swears by the sport, but I just don't think it's humane. A good coon fight, now that's something different."

When we had finished getting the dressing over the splint, I told Coon to take Bear on home but bring him back to see me by the end of the week. Bear made four return trips for redressing and treatment before the splint was removed, but he did make an excellent recovery.

Late that summer Coon drove up to the office in his pickup, stopped, got out, and came in. My station wagon was outside so he knew I was there.

"Junior, Bear has got another problem."

"What's it this time, Coon?"

"He's paralyzed. Can't hardly move a muscle. Been that way for two days now. Keeps getting worse. Thought I better bring him by."

"Glad to take a look. Is he out in the pickup?"

"Yes, he's laying on some burlap sacks in the rear end. I'll bring him on in."

A few minutes later Bear was stretched out on the floor of the office, He could blink his eyelids but move very little else. As Coon had said, Bear was paralyzed.

"Think he got ahold of something to get poisoned on, Junior?"

"I don't think so, but let me examine him."

I ran my hands over his body surface and found what I was looking for. A tick was embedded on the upper neck area just back of the skull. Its body was engorged with blood. A pledget of cotton saturated with alcohol was enough to intoxicate the tick so it released its grasp sufficiently for me to remove it with tweezers. "There's your trouble, Coon. Those ticks secrete a toxin that can cause paralysis. Bear should be all right now."

"But, Junior, I've had ticks all over me and never been paralyzed. I think Jennie would wish I'd get paralyzed when I come to bed some nights. I don't think she begrudges me those nights hunting at all."

"Well, Coon, if you got one of those ticks at the base of your skull like Bear here, you could get paralyzed."

"Junior, you're quite a vet. Armer taught you well. Belle has a new litter out at the farm. You need some special honoring. I'm going to name the big male in that litter, Junior. He's out of Bear, so he ought to be quite a dog. All the county is going to know about Junior after I get through training him with Bear. You're going to have a famous namesake. Isn't that wonderful, Junior?"

I agreed that it was wonderful, wanting to be diplomatic. Somehow, I had never looked with wholehearted favor on the name Junior and had gone by the names James or Jimmy when I went away to college.

When I went home for dinner I told Marian, "Marian, if we have a boy we won't be able to name him after Armer and me."

"I didn't know you wanted to, but why not?" Marian asked.

"Well, Coon Maxwell is showing his gratitude for my service by naming the pick of Belle's litter for me, so you see, the name is taken."

"You need to copyright that name if it is going to be that popular."

"That may be right. How much do you suppose I could get for patent rights to my name?"

"That depends on how many animals you make well, evidently."

"It might be more profitable just to collect some of the money owed by those farmers."

"Now, you're getting your feet back on the ground. I hope Coon isn't paying Bear's vet bills by naming animals after you."

"Now, Marian, you know that isn't so." Just then the telephone rang, interrupting Marian's reply.

"Can We Feed 2,000 People?"

THE county fair is the event of the year for rural America. A blue ribbon won for an exhibit of a jar of pickles is as prized as a diploma earned for graduating from grade school. The prize for grand champion steer will occupy a prominent place on the mantel of the recipient for the remainder of his life. Row upon row of buildings filled with exhibits of the culinary arts, of sewing, of the fine arts, of crops, of livestock, and of the commercial suppliers to the agricultural field attest to the widespread interest in the event. Of even more importance to those not talented enough to compete for ribbons is the opportunity to take in the carnival with its rides and sideshow attractions and to take in the entertainment—the rodeos, the races, the pulling contests—or the other events that are the highlights of each fair.

For many years Fredonia, Kansas, hosted the Wilson County Fair, which was noted throughout the Middle West for harness racing. In 1930 it was discontinued. Although many of us were youngsters at that time, the excitement of fair days and of horse racing lingered on in our memories.

I remember being taken by my Grandfather Short, while I was still a preschool child, to see the fair. I was impatient to go on the rides, but Grandfather insisted on first going through the exhibit buildings. In the building housing the baked goods, he spotted a plate of cookies with a blue ribbon beside it.

"Those cookies were baked by May Ogden. She was your Sunday School teacher when you were in the nursery class."

"Can I have a cooky, Grandpa?" I had no recollection of May Ogden, but the cookies looked good.

"No, these are for exhibit. Only the judges get to eat these. Maybe I can get her to bake you a batch of cookies later on. I'll talk to her when she comes into the store for groceries Saturday."

I didn't want cookies later. I wanted one now but it was useless to argue with Grandfather Short when he said "No!" I decided I was going to be a cooky judge when I grew up. Although I've never yet qualified, I'm still sampling cookies, hoping to attain this childhood ambition.

Later, in the cattle barn, we saw a steer with the Grand Champion blue ribbon pinned to its head board.

"See that fine looking steer, Junior? The name card says it belongs to Mary Smith. I think that's Bert's daughter. I bet that Bert is proud as punch of Mary."

Still later, when he finally guided me to the midway of the carnival, I was attracted by the spiel of the barker at one of the sideshows.

"Come on over, ladies and gentlemen. Step right up. I'm not going to bite you. Step up front here. Hey, Grampa, come on over." He was hollering in Grandfather's direction. Grandfather tried to ignore him. "I've got something over here that'll make you feel twenty years younger." Addressing the growing crowd, "I'm here to introduce you to six of the seven marvels of the modern world. The only reason I can't introduce you to the seventh is because the eighty-six-year-old tattooed lady, Mrs. Bessy, is having to take time out to have a baby. Yes sir, this is her sixth child since she was sixty. The doctors up at Harvard spent two days examining Bessy last month and pronounced her normal in every way. They were astounded at her fertility at that advanced age. Bessy can't be with us today but promises to be back next year with her bouncing baby if she isn't pregnant again."

"What's he talking about, Grandpa?"

"Don't pay any attention to that trash, Junior. Would you like to go on the merry-go-round?"

"Don't be afraid. Come up here to the front. You over there in the yellow shirt, step over here. Don't be bashful. I'm not going to bite. That's it. Come on up closer so you can see what made 678 men file for divorce. I'm going to bring out Lizzie, the snake charmer. Lizzie is more than just a snake charmer as you'll soon see. Come on out Lizzie. All right, ladies and gentlemen, give her a hand."

Lizzie, an excessively rouged platinum blonde, appeared wearing a worn blue bathrobe gaping open at the top, exposing her pendulous breasts barely confined by a bandana handerchief bra.

"Yes, sir, Lizzie defies death several times a day by entering our snake pit inside and exposing herself to the most deadly vipers the world has ever seen, collected into one pit. Yes sir, one drop of their venom will send a person to the Pearly Gates in thirty seconds, but Lizzie charms these snakes. She wraps them around her neck, she allows them to crawl over her body, she does things with these vipers that no other person has ever done. She has also charmed men with her extrasensory powers. So mama, hang on to your men when you step up here to buy a ticket."

"Grandpa, can I see the snake charmer?"

Grandfather Short didn't answer. He was trying to attract me out of earshot of the barker before I heard something unfit for my ears. "Junior, how about going on the Ferris wheel? It's down at the other end of the midway."

"Oh boy! Yes! Yes! Will you take me, Grandpa?"

Later, from the top of the Ferris wheel, we looked out over the crowds and the buildings. Over to the left we could see the horses running heats around the racetrack. The roar of the crowds, in the grandstand and along the track fence urging their favorites to victory, reached us above the noise of the carnival. It was a sensational experience for a youth.

Years later, in the fifties, an effort was being made to reactivate the county fair. It was to be held in conjunction with the annual 4-H exhibition. Only one building remained of the former set of exhibit buildings. A few years previously, the 4-H fathers had constructed a pole building to house livestock. These two buildings, an allotment from a county tax fund, and nostalgia were all the promoters had to go on. They begged exhibit space in empty buildings around town. They planned entertainment that could be presented with minimal funding, again in areas scattered around town. The crowds were dispersed, growth income was minimal, and the group faced insurmountable obstacles.

My new office was on the edge of the former fairgrounds. I observed the activities taking place there and compared them with the visions I had of the fair of twenty-five years previous. Before my eyes were two exhibit buildings. In former years there were eight or more buildings. Also, there had been a grandstand, a half-mile racetrack, and dozens of stables for the horses.

When Joe Hardy, the Wilson County Fair president, was in the area I would render my unsolicited advice on how to develop the fair. Joe responded to my advice by adroitly, without my foreknowlege, promoting my election as president of the Wilson County Fair at the next annual meeting. I did not know my name was to be offered and had left town to visit relatives. I wasn't there to protest, so I became president.

Like conceiving a baby, criticism is easy. It is far more difficult to deliver. I had asked for it by my criticism, now I was expected to deliver. Actually, no one person can deliver on a project of this magnitude. One of the primary purposes of a leader is to enthuse others to work. In this case there were many persons like myself who were eager to see the fair reactivated. It was not difficult to generate the enthusiasm. My objective was to channel this enthusiasm into productive outlets.

The board of directors agreed that the lack of money should not be a limiting factor. We would find the money. It was also agreed that somehow, if we were to succeed, we would have to centralize the fair at the fairgrounds. Furthermore, to draw the crowds necessary to put the fair on the road to success, we would have to present top-flight entertainment. We would have to get additional covered space within the fairgrounds.

To centralize the fair, we arranged to borrow tents from the National Guard. For entertainment, it was decided to feature an afternoon of horse racing on the former racetrack. The track would be regraded, a starting gate would be borrowed from a neighboring fair, and snow fencing borrowed from the highway department could be used to fence the track. We hoped it would be a major attraction. To insure its attractiveness, we decided to present it and all other entertainment free. We would have a "free" fair. However, we were still doubtful of our ability to attract a crowd. If we could attract two thousand persons to the grounds during the fair days, we were on the way. If we only attracted one thousand, we were doomed. To insure attendance, we decided to have a barbecue one evening and feed all present free. We were completely naive about the entertainment business; we had no conception of what we were letting ourselves in for.

The cost alone was a disturbing factor. We were obligating ourselves for several thousands of dollars. How were we going to raise the money if the entertainment and barbecue were free? The tax allotment could not be used for other than exhibit purposes and would have been inadequate in any case. The carnival would generate only limited funds. Rental income from commercial exhibits would be minimal. Membership dues helped, but nobody would be apt to make donations of significant amounts. We needed an "angel." The suggestion was made that we sell advertisement space in a fair program book. If we could raise twenty-five hundred dollars by that method, we were on the way.

But, could we raise that amount? Twenty-five hundred dollars was still a lot of money in the fifties. I was experienced in selling services; I knew nothing of the art of selling advertisement space. To me, twenty-five hundred dollars was a lot of money to raise by that method. I had not yet been exposed to the "boiler room" tactics of salesmen for real estate, for commodities, or for donations to police benevolent associations. All that was to come years later.

Fortunately, we had a person in our midst who could have put the "boiler room" salesmen who contacted me in later years to shame. If she had put her mind to larceny through telephone solicitation, she could have gotten enough money to have bought her own private South Seas island and retired to it at an early age. However, she chose to remain honest. She became a dedicated booster for the fair and, like the rest of us, donated her services to the cause. Her seductive voice over the telephone charmed many a hard-headed businessman who had heard not a kind word from his wife in many a year. Ellen Johnson contributed as much with her persuasive telephone manner to the success of the Wilson County Fair as the rest of us contributed with our physical efforts. Ellen raised the money necessary for us to proceed.

One of the major undertakings we faced was preparing to feed a barbecue dinner to an unknown number of people. From the standpoint that it was free, the persons to be fed should have had no reason to complain. From the standpoint of whether we would ever attract a crowd to a future fair, it was essential that the barbecue dinner be adequate and well received by all who attended. How many persons should we plan to feed? How much food would it take? How did one go about preparing a barbecue for two thousand persons? Ellen raised the money to get us started. Our success now depended on how we answered the preceding questions.

We prepared for two thousand persons. Sitting in Miami, Florida, as I write, that figure seems ridiculous. A fire in a warehouse down on the highway would attract that many here. However, Fredonia was a different world. Not since the fair with its harness racing some thirty years before, had Fredonia seen crowds of that magnitude at the fair grounds. A Santa Claus parade or a Homecoming Day parade uptown might attract a few thousand persons. Could free entertainment and a barbecue attract a sizeable number to the park? We needed two thousand. Four thousand would stretch our resources. Ten thousand would be just as catastrophic as one thousand.

We solicited advice on quantities of food and methods of preparation from persons at a neighboring county fair experienced in this field—although they had never been so foolhardy as to undertake to serve the food free. But then they were established; they weren't desperately trying to get started. Furthermore, they didn't have an Ellen with her sultry voice to separate the merchants from their money so couldn't have gone our route if they wished.

"Dutch" Kelsey, a local butcher, was in charge of the meat preparation. One ton of beef was purchased—I am referring to processed beef, not beef on the hoof. With this, Dutch was expected to repeat the miracle of the loaves and the fishes if need be. The meat was cut into seven-pound chunks, sprinkled with seasoning, wrapped, and placed into a cooler. Dutch made arrangements to purchase the necessary beans, bread, chips, and drinks that were needed to complete the meals.

"Hedgewood" was used to cook the meat. This meant that several truckloads of the wood had to be collected from around the county by volunteers and hauled to the area where the barbecue pit was to be dug. A pit six-feet deep, four-feet wide, and ten-feet long was dug. Forty-eight hours before serving time, the pit was filled with wood and set ablaze. Our advisors from the neighboring county volunteered their services in tending the fire in return for sufficient liquid refreshment. Dutch advised us to grab their offer.

"Hell, Doc, I'm not up to that all-night drinking anymore. Besides, Louise isn't used to being without a bed partner."

The liquor was provided to the all-night fire tenders and after sharing a few spiked cokes with them, we left them to their duties. After twenty-four hours, a bed of coals fifteen-inches deep covered the pit floor. This was then leveled and covered with four inches of sand. The chunks of meat were hauled to the pit site and carefully distributed on the hot sandy floor by volunteers willing to suffer "hot feet." After the "hot-footed" men were helped from the pit, it was first covered with metal boiler plate and then with a mound of dirt, creating an airtight oven.

A ton of beef and the future of our fair laid buried in the hole in the ground. I had never before been involved in preparing meat in this fashion. Would the meat be ready when we opened the pit twenty-four hours later? We hoped we would have a crowd to feed. We had to have the meat ready to go. Needless to say, I was uneasy. Dutch assured me everything would be O.K.

"Doc, you get the people here; I'll have the food ready."

I was still skeptical. That night I slept fitfully. About 2:00 A.M. I arose, dressed, and drove to the fairgrounds. The dirt covering the oven was warm. Nobody was around. Our fire tenders were probably catching up on sleep lost from tending the fire of the previous night. I drove back to my house, undressed, and got back in bed beside Marian.

"Where have you been, Jim?"

"Out seeing about a cow."

She grunted and went back to sleep. I couldn't relax and go back to sleep. For the next hours I tossed and turned. When daybreak came, I arose and went downstairs to prepare coffee. The day dawned bright and warm. It was a typical August day for Kansas. I drank a cup of coffee and tried to concentrate on reading yesterday's newspaper. Sometime later, Marian joined me and prepared breakfast.

"Where did you go last night?"

"Down to the fairgrounds."

"Why? Didn't you get enough to drink the night before?"

I grunted and changed the subject. She wouldn't have understood anyway.

After breakfast I drove to my office. It had been converted into the headquarters office for the fair. The morning was spent checking in the exhibits. The people, though enthusiastic, were not numerous. I nervously began to wonder if I had overestimated the drawing attraction of free races and barbecue.

By 11:00 A.M. the judging of the home economics projects was underway. Young 4-H girls and a few older ladies came by smilingly displaying their ribbons. The last of the livestock was being unloaded and assigned stall space. Their judging wouldn't commence until the next day. A few horse trailers pulled into the park and unloaded horses in preparation for the races that afternoon. At least we would have races, even if few were there to witness them. I could look out across the fairgrounds from my front door and nearly count the number of people. A carnival was just opening up but barely a dozen persons were waiting to storm the midway. I shrugged my shoulders and went back inside. At least we had tried.

I need not have worried. Shortly after noon cars began streaming into the fairgrounds. Extra police were found to assist in orderly parking. By 1:00 P.M., an hour before race time, every vacant space in the park was filled with cars. Others were being forced to park outside and the occupants had to walk a few blocks to gain entrance. Such a crowd hadn't been seen in Fredonia for years. At race time, under a blistering sun, thousands crowded the track fences loudly encouraging their favorite horses and jockeys as they broke from the starting gate and thundered down the track. The races were an astounding success.

The time to feed the multitude finally arrived. Serving tables had been set up. The beans, coleslaw, bread, chips, catsup, pickles, coffee, cold drinks, and the cups, paper plates, napkins, plastic eating utensils were distributed at their appropriate places. The members of the local Rotary and Lions clubs were present to assist in the serving. All was in readiness but the meat. Was it cooked?

We could wait no longer so a crew was sent over to uncover the pit and retrieve the packages of meat.

"What do you think, Dutch? Is it ready?"

"Don't worry, Doc. It's ready."

True to his word the meat, when unpacked, proved to be delicious. The serving lines rapidly dispensed the food to the waiting lines of people. Card tables, folding chairs, blankets, and other sundry picnic furniture appeared out of cars. Soon the park was a vast picnic ground. We would have run out of food except that many persons left after the races, presuming that there would not be enough food or that it would take too long to serve. Even then we served nearly three thousand persons.

"Doc, I told you we would feed them if you got them here." Dutch was relaxing on the tailgate of the pickup used to haul the meat, nursing a spiked coke.

"You did, didn't you? Where did you get the booze? I thought you used the last of it the other night to supply our fire tenders."

"Oh, Charley made another run over to Joplin. Couldn't have horse racing without some cheer, now could we?"

Conversation drifted to recapitulating the races of the afternoon. "Did you see young Simmons bring that sorrel of Packer's out that gate? He was half-way down the track before the others were out the gate."

All the races were rerun while accepting congratulations for the excellent barbecue from the recipients. All of us were happy and the persons imbibing the shipment from Joplin were happier yet. The fair, no matter what happened the next couple of days, was a success.

That night, as I slipped into bed beside Marian, I heard her inquire. "Are you going to have to see about a cow tonight?"

I just grunted. Two minutes later I was sound asleep.

"Coming Out of Gate Four on Calamity Jane . . ."

THE Wilson County Free Fair of 1958 was an outstanding success. However, major problems remained to be solved before the fair was on a firm footing. The most serious was securing adequate funds to construct exhibit buildings and entertainment facilities. It required labor to haul tents for housing, for exhibits, and for snow fencing to line the racetrack at the fairgrounds. It required labor to erect the tents and snow fencing. It required still more labor to take these structures down and return them to where they came from. All of this could be done one year with volunteer labor. It could not be done year after year with such labor. There is a limit to how long one's enthusiasm can be maintained.

Another problem that arose from erecting tents for housing swine on a dirt surface was that of hog wallows with the attendant malodorous condition. Swine had to be kept cool by sprinkling them when hot—and it did get hot under canvas in Kansas in August. A must was an exhibit building with a concrete floor for the swine. Other exhibit buildings, while needed, were put at a lower priority.

Annually, we could get limited funding for exhibit buildings from tax sources under a law we found on the statutes. Tax funding, however, was not available for recreational facilities. This funding had to come from other sources, but these facilities would generate income that could be used for expansion. We were stumped on how to proceed. We needed an "angle" or we needed to hold a lot of "pie suppers." For some two months after the fair, we basked in the glory of success and debated about how to proceed. We might have remained forever at this point if it hadn't been for the intervention of a person who volunteered to lead a fund-raising program for us.

This person, Ben Laidlow, telephoned and requested that I stop by his home one Sunday morning. I had no idea what the meeting was for but courtesy and curiosity prompted me to accept the invitation. When I arrived at his house, he invited me in and settled me in an easy chair with a bourbon and soda. Ben complimented our group on our efforts in making the previous fair a success. He suggested that the county fair and the Fredonia homecoming celebration ought to be combined to make one of the largest events in that part of Kansas. He may have been right but they were two different events, for different groups, and with different leaders. That idea never got off the ground. He further suggested that a fund-raising drive be undertaken to get the money needed to build the fair facilities.

"Dr. Porter, how much money do you need?" He practiced professional courtesy and didn't call me Doc.

"Well, Ben, we've got to have bleachers and we need some structural facilities for the entertainment. The cost of the latter will depend upon the type of entertainment decided on."

"What type of entertainment are you considering? Racing?"

"Yes, this is one type of entertainment we are considering but we are faced with the fact that the space occupied by the former one-half mile racetrack isn't intact. The livestock sales barn now occupies the north turn of that track. We can move the track south but that is going to take a lot of grading and some rerouting of present roads. Besides, harness racing, if we hold that type of racing, is an expensive sport. We have to guarantee a lot of money. One or two rainy days could bankrupt us."

"Insurance can protect you from a rain washout."

"That's probably right; but the profit to be made on that type of entertainment, considering the prize money that has to be guaranteed, is minimal. We need something we can stage cheaper from which to net more money. We need money, not prestige!"

"There's going to be some unhappy persons around Fredonia if you don't go to harness racing, but what are the alternatives?"

"Some of us were talking about an amateur rodeo. The participants pay entry fees. We would have to put up added money to attract good cowboys, but our costs would be far below that of staging harness racing. We should come out far better financially."

"What about horse racing or team pulling or some of these other events?"

"All of them have potential, but I think a good amateur rodeo will draw more and profit us more in the long run."

"Well, your group is going to have to decide on the answer to that. If you do decide on a rodeo, what will you have to construct and what will the costs be?"

"We need bleachers. That will cost a few thousand. However, they do have a set of bleachers at a defunct car track south of Neodesha that might be for sale. They are just sitting there rusting and rotting away. We might be able to purchase those on time."

"They do have the one grandstand left in the fairground. People use it for softball games held there."

"Yes, that's right. If we have a rodeo, we will have to move the grandstand, but that can be done."

"How much seating will that give you?"

"If we get the bleachers from Neodesha or construct the equivalent and take over the present grandstand, we ought to be able to seat two thousand. There are always five hundred to one thousand persons who want to sit on baled hay along the arena fencing, so we could make out on that."

"Bleachers can be rented, can't they? It seems like Eureka rented bleachers for their harness racing."

"Certainly, but again this begins to cut into costs."

"O.K. What else do you need—lights, chutes, pens—what else?"

"We can probably make arrangements to buy the present lights used for softball from the city. That will take care of that problem if they'll give us terms not to pay until after the rodeo."

"They'll do that."

"We will have to construct pens and chutes and fence the arena. That will take up to one thousand dollars for materials plus a lot of volunteer labor."

"Volunteer labor seems to be your strong suit. O.K. How much money would you make on a three-night rodeo?"

"I presume we ought to net twenty-five hundred dollars the first year."

"All right, if you had twenty-five hundred dollars now to work with and were expecting to make twenty-five hundred dollars from the rodeo, could you get the necessary facilities constructed and stage the rodeo?"

"Of course we could," I said without hesitation. Ben must be dreaming. Where would we get twenty-five hundred dollars?

"Then I'll see that the twenty-five hundred dollars is provided."

Ben proposed heading a fund-raising drive to raise the money by soliciting one hundred persons to contribute twenty-five dollars each. To me this idea seemed preposterous. I had considerable trepidation about our being able to get five or ten dollars each from local businessmen for ads in our fair book. At least there they were getting something of nominal value for the expense. Here they were getting nothing. True, the construction of most of the churches in Fredonia had been financed by contributions. There, though, they took deductions on income tax reports and would get credit in the ledger that St. Peter kept at the Pearly Gates. The county fair couldn't offer those inducements. It was also true the local hospital had been built because sufficient funds were raised by donations to match available federal funds. But again these donations were deductible from income taxes and there was a difference between a seat at a rodeo and a bed in a hospital.

I was skeptical but Ben had gauged the community's attitude far better than I. I was on the inside and didn't fully trust the public adoration that was being radiated in our direction. Ben was on the outside and knew, because of our success of the previous summer, that the local people were enthusiastic about the possibility of a fair and would contribute the necessary funding to get it started. Ben was right and the money was raised.

It did take some persuasion to get all the active workers to agree on a rodeo. One or two persons had strong desires to stage harness racing as in the days of yore. Fredonia had been known throughout the Middle West in those days because it was on the harness track circuit. Eureka, Winfield, and other Kansas towns were still staging harness racing. Why couldn't Fredonia? It came down to money. We needed money to get started.

The prestige of staging harness racing didn't outweigh the pragmatic consideration of needing money. After a few weeks of debate among ourselves, a consensus was reached that the Wilson County Fair would promote an amateur rodeo.

That winter a contract was signed with a rodeo promoter to furnish livestock for the show. Not one post had been set for the pens or chutes, but we were optimistic that everything would be ready. We negotiated with the city for the purchase, on contract, of the floodlights and the grandstand at the softball field. We would construct our rodeo arena where the softball field had been. Because of the severe weather during the winter and planting activities during the spring, very little else was done until June arrived. We had two months left to erect our facilities. A newly graduated veterinarian, Dr. Jim Smart, joined me in my practice. Dr. Armer, my father, had retired to sales barn and meat inspection work. Dr. Smart managed the practice while I supervised the construction work.

I had been making preliminary plans for the construction so we lost no time once we started. A truckload of two-by-four lumber had been purchased and hauled in from a sawmill in Arkansas. For this we had to pay cash—some five hundred dollars. I got the city to donate discarded lampposts that were sawed into the proper length and used for the upright posts on the chutes and pens. We were able to purchase the three hundred feet of bleachers from the defunct auto track some twenty miles away—again on time. I arranged to purchase every bolt, six inches or longer, in town on credit to bolt together the pens and chutes. I designed, with the advice of several of the local rodeo cowboys, a set of pens with a calf chute and featuring six bucking chutes for the bucking broncos and the bulls. Overlooking these chutes was an official and dignitary stand capable of seating some one hundred persons.

One hot day in late spring a crew of volunteers was assembled to aid a couple of truckers who had volunteered their services and flatbed trucks to haul the bleachers to the future rodeo grounds. One group used saws and torches to cut the bleachers into fifteen-foot lengths. The remainder of the volunteers divided up into two groups, one to work with each truck. Work started early in the morning. Every half-hour until late in the afternoon a truck would pull into the rodeo grounds and the crew would unload another section of bleachers. By evening we had bleachers, lumber, telephone posts, and practically all of our needed materials lying around the grounds. Everything was ready for the construction of the rodeo facilities.

In early June, two months before the fair, a heavy rain caused a flash flood from a nearby creek that swept away all our lumber. When the water started receding, we waded in to survey our losses. The lumber was indeed washed away but the other materials—the bleachers and the posts—were still there. We didn't have the time or the money to go after another truckload of lumber.

"Well, Doc, it was a good try anyway," said Dutch. "I was looking forward to seeing the Webb boys perform though."

"I guess we could feature a pulling contest. We still have the bleachers," I commented.

"Doc, suppose we could sell the telephone posts to somebody to get a little prize money for the teamsters?"

"You fellows may be overly pessimistic. It's two miles to the river. Some of the lumber may be stranded between here and there. Bill and I are going to take a look this afternoon," Dave volunteered.

Late that evening Dave reported back that practically all the lumber had been miraculously stranded before reaching the river. We were still in business. Two or three days were lost while volunteers waded or muddled into fields along the watercourse and lugged out to dry-land trucks a piece of lumber at a time. Dave was right, miraculously the lumber was all there.

We had lost another week though. Barely seven weeks remained until fair time and nothing had been constructed. A call went out for volunteers. During the day two or three men might be helping me at the grounds. By night, under the floodlights, a dozen or more men would be working. The posts were set, siding was bolted to the upright posts, chute gates were bolted together and hung. Little by little, week by week, we began to make progress. Dr. Jim Smart, my associate veterinarian, managed the practice; I became a rodeo facility construction foreman. My family seldom saw me; my clients never saw me unless they worked as volunteers.

A month before the fair, another catastrophe struck. Another heavy rain occurred and a record flood swept through the grounds. This time we had warning and took precautions. We waded into the area, even as the water was rising around our legs, and tied all loose lumber to upright posts or to the bleachers. When the floodwaters receded two days later, we found we had lost nothing except time.

Since little more than three weeks remained, efforts were redoubled. Volunteers worked all day in their fields and then came in at night to help bolt the rodeo facilities together, to get the arena fencing up, to get skids welded under the bleachers, and later to paint them. A group of the 4-H fathers found time to lay a concrete platform and erect a pole building over it for housing the swine. The barbecue crew cut up and packaged the meat and hauled in the lumber needed for the pit.

Somehow, everything was ready for the fair and rodeo in spite of having been without funds scarcely six months before and in spite of having experienced two floods that had inundated the grounds. The first day of the fair found the buildings and tents crammed with exhibits. The carnival was set up and ready to operate. Rodeo stock had been hauled in and unloaded into the pens. Amateur cowboys appeared from a four-state area and paid entry fees to participate. We did put up a sizable amount of added purse money to attract quality. Earlier, we had decided to go with an amateur rodeo rather than a professional RCA (Rodeo Cowboys of America) rodeo. As with the harness racing, the prestige of having a professional rodeo wasn't justified, given our financial circumstances.

The barbecue was furnished free to the crowd the first night immediately before the rodeo. Fully five thousand persons were fed in less than two hours. Again, the food was delicious and the people were pleased. Now remained the rodeo.

None of us had any previous experience in managing a rodeo. I had attended a few rodeos during the summer, including the professional rodeo at Nowata, Oklahoma, the cowboy capital of the world, just to sharpen up on what was to occur. We got Ellen Johnson, our "boiler room" solicitor, to manage the entry books. She had never seen a rodeo although she had lived in cattle country all her life. She was fascinated by the task and thought some of the young cowboys really looked cute and innocent. Since we were financially embarrassed, volunteers manned all the official posts. I was the announcer and sat up in the dignitary stands above the chutes trying to keep a running commentary going to the crowd about what was occurring in the chutes underneath and in the arena after the broncs or bulls were released. The announcer and the rodeo clown(s) were supposed to keep the show strung together and the audience entertained between events. The clown had the added task of protecting thrown cowboys from the plunging and angry bulls and broncs. Many a cowboy owes his health to the fearlessness of these unsung heroes, the clowns. Also, the clowns always had a string of jokes, some slightly earthy, which the announcer had to help them deliver. The announcer was supposed to be the fall guy and would parrot back the desired answers to the clown's questions until the clown delivered the punch line and the audience would roar at the announcer's faked embarrassment. We also had volunteer judges and timers from our local group, a situation that was to cause us serious problems the next night.

Everything went smoothly the first night as far as I could tell, sitting up in my "catbird's nest."

"Here out of gate four comes Jim Snyder on Calamity Jane. Jim has won prize money in ten of the twelve rodeos he has participated in this summer. Jim has paid his money just like all the others, but tonight he may be contributing to his opponents because he drew Calamity Jane. Nobody has managed to stay on Calamity Jane for the required eight seconds yet this summer. Calamity Jane just doesn't like to have those cowboys on top of her. Yes sir, she sure is kicking up down there in chute four. Jim has tried to get down on top of her bare back twice now and has had to come right back up twice. Calamity Jane just doesn't want anything to do with him. Whoa there, girl!

Easy does it! There, Jim Snyder is easing down on her back again. Now he has his hand strap held tight in his hand. Ready! Ready! Jim nods his head. The gate is swinging open. Here she comes."

She bucks, she twists, she kicks; Jim whoops, he spurs, he swings his free hand. Two seconds, three seconds—each second seems an eternity to a person on a bucking bronc. Four seconds, Calamity Jane twists to the right and jackknifes her back. Jim can stay on no longer and goes sailing through the air. The clown appears at his side instantly and two mounted cowboys hem the bronc in and direct her away from the dislodged rider. One of the mounted cowboys reaches over and unloosens the bucking cinch.

Event after event was run off: the saddle bronc, the calf roping, the bareback bronc, the bulldogging, the bull riding—the latter said to be the most dangerous event of all. Finally, the evening was over and we congratulated ourselves on a job well done—congratulations that were premature as it turned out.

The second night the opening ceremony had taken place in which many cowgirls and cowboys in fanciful costumes paraded into the arena. My colleague, Jim Smart, sang the "Star Spangled Banner." The riders left the arena. The saddle bronc riding was ready to begin. The horses were in the chutes. Dan Blake was supposed to be coming out of gate three on Black Thunder—but no Dan. We had heard rumors that the cowboys were displeased with our judges. They didn't think them competent. If they couldn't pick their judges, there would be no rodeo. However, they paid their entry fees. Contestants had never chosen their judges. We figured it was all bluff. There had never been a strike at an amateur rodeo yet. We didn't expect that Fredonia would have the honor of being the first town to be the victim of a rodeo strike. Besides, we had local volunteers to ride if the regular cowboys wouldn't ride. True, the cowboys had paid entry fees for those horses, but we arranged to have a second string of broncs ready for our volunteer riders that hadn't been paid for.

The audience was unaware of what was transpiring. I was keeping up a running commentary as if Dan Blake was having trouble settling into the saddle on Black Thunder—but no Dan. Dan and his cohorts were back of the chutes engaged in heated discussions with my colleagues. They would select their judges or there would be no rodeo.

"To hell with that! This is our rodeo! If you don't want to participate, get out. We have another string of livestock and volunteer cowboys ready to go."

"Nobody rides if we don't."

"Who says so?"

"You're looking at who says so."

"Bill, get ready to mount if Dan doesn't want to ride."

"If Bill mounts, both he and his saddle are going to come off once the chute gate is opened."

"Hell, what do you want? We have experienced judges."

"Like hell they are. We'll pick our own judges from among the entries not entered in the particular event."

The threat of violence, the mention of saddles coming un cinched, was enough to sober my colleagues. The conversations became more conciliatory.

In the meantime I was trying to maintain the audience's suspense while describing the imaginary problems Dan was having trying to mount Black Thunder. The clown, sensing my problems, released a goat into the arena and demonstrated his ability to run down and bulldog the protesting "Billy."

Meanwhile, back of the chutes, my colleagues decided to accept the terms of the strikers. Word was sent to me. Would I agree to the capitulation? The crowd was getting impatient. The clown's antics with the billy goat were beginning to pale. The show had to go on. I agreed to the capitulation. The strikers quickly chose judges from their midst and the rodeo went on. The audience never realized that they had been present at a rodeo strike.

The fair again proved successful. While expenses for construction had run higher than expected, we were able to finance our debts on the strength of a successful rodeo. In succeeding years the fair officers required that the rodeo stock contractor provide the rodeo judges. In the succeeding years, because of the popularity of the barbecue, the food was placed within the gates of the rodeo arena so that a ticket to the rodeo was required before a person was fed. The fair continued to grow year after year due to the enthusiasm of the Wilson County Fair Association members.

I left Fredonia to return to graduate school after this fair and did not return at fair time until some seven years later. During those intervening years I traveled many miles and had many experiences. However, in all of my travels I never met a group of persons more dedicated to a goal than the members of that fair association. At the time of my return, a building was dedicated in my honor—the James A. Porter, Jr., Building. My father, Armer, died that same day, symbolizing the passing of an era. In my remarks at the ceremony I spoke glowingly of the quality of the people in the area—the children and grandchildren of persons who had homesteaded and developed the area after the Civil War. As long as our nation is composed of individuals who, to paraphrase John F. Kennedy, ask not what your country can do for you, but what you can do for your country, our country will continue to be a great nation.

Wags Has Worms

ZOONOSES are diseases transmitted from animals to man. Rabies is one of the best known because of the death that nearly always results in infected persons. This is the reason that dogs and cats should be vaccinated at periodic intervals. There are a hundred or more other zoonotic diseases. Undulant fever is an occupational disease of veterinarians due to contact with cows or swine infected with brucellosis. It was one of the diseases from which I periodically suffered while in practice. Ringworm is another disease that children often get from intimate contact with infected dogs and cats.

Not all diseases transmitted from animals to man are harmful. Cowpox transmitted to milkers' hands resulted in an immunity to smallpox. This led to Jenner's development of smallpox vaccine.

Other infections occasionally occurred in man or in animals that were not transmittable but could cause emotional problems. This was the situation that I confronted with Virginia Allen.

Virginia, matronly and middle-aged, was an emotional and/or hysterical woman. The sight of a mouse would find her climbing furniture and screaming. The sight of a cockroach would keep her spraying and cleaning cupboards for weeks on end. The sight of a flea would find her buying every brand of flea powder or spray available in town to use on Wags, her blonde, female cocker spaniel.

One morning the telephone at my home rang while I was still eating breakfast. I answered and found myself talking to Virginia Allen.

"Dr. Porter, this is Virginia Allen."

"Yes, Mrs. Allen, what can I do for you?"

"I'm going to send my husband, Carl, down to your office with Wags. You're going to have to put her to sleep."

"You mean kill her? For what reason?"

"I can't talk about it."

"Well, Mrs. Allen, surely that flea infestation she had shouldn't justify killing her."

"No, that's not it."

"Well, what is it? Maybe I can help."

"I'm really too embarrassed to say anything."

"Now, Mrs. Allen. I don't embarrass easily and this is my business. What is wrong with Wags?"

"Dr. Porter, I'll tell you but you musn't ever tell anybody. It would be so embarrassing to me. Promise?"

"Certainly. Now please tell me what is Wags' problem?"

"Wags has worms, Dr. Porter. It is horrible."

"Mrs. Allen, lots of dogs have worms. That is not horrible because worms can be treated."

"Dr. Porter, you don't understand. It isn't just Wags. My baby, Barbara, has worms, too. She caught them from Wags. It's awful. I don't want to think about it, but I just can't keep the dog around to keep infecting Barbara."

"Mrs. Allen, most worms of dogs don't infect people directly. How do you know Barbara has worms?"

"Dr. Porter, it's embarrassing. I really can't talk about it but she does have worms."

"Mrs. Allen, you're asking me to kill Wags. You do like the dog. I'm not embarrassed by these things. This is my business. Please tell me how you know Barbara has worms?"

"Dr. Porter, I saw worms. They were squirming all over her bowel movement. It was horrible. I can't stand to have worms in my house. I'll get Barbara treated by Dr. Mitchell, but you've got to put Wags to sleep. I can't go through this again."

"Now, Mrs. Allen, were these small threadlike, white worms?"

"Yes, Dr. Porter."

"Mrs. Allen, those are probably pinworms. They are parasites of human beings. They are not parasites of dogs."

"Oh, Dr. Porter. The Allens don't have worms. The worms must have come from Wags."

"I'm sorry, but the Allens or some persons close to them do have pinworms if the worms are really pinworms. Wags doesn't have pinworms."

"Dr. Porter, are you saying that Carl or I gave the infection to Barbara? How could you suggest such a thing?"

"Look, Mrs. Allen, have Carl bring a stool sample from Wags to my office. Have Dr. Mitchell check Barbara. Let's wait until we check things out."

"Well, if you say so, Dr. Porter. But I'm frantic. Carl will be right down to your office." She hung up.

American society, through the utilization of sanitary sewers and the wearing of shoes, has separated itself from most parasites. Pinworms, however, have proven themselves fully capable of living in an affluent society. The eggs are practically ubiquitous in houses where there are children until the age they are toilet trained. This is the one parasite for which pharmaceutical companies are willing to invest money in marketing a drug. It strikes the children of the affluent, it is practically cosmopolitan, and it is a money maker.

Carl did bring a stool sample to my office. It was negative. Dr. Mitchell calmed Virginia down and gave her a prescription plus directions for household sanitation. Wags was accepted back into the good graces of the Allen family.

One day, the following December, I returned home for dinner.

"Jim, you've got a Christmas card from Wags Allen. Who's Wags Allen?"

"Wags? Oh, that must be Virginia's dog."

"Virginia. I'd better see what this says."

She opened and read the card. "Jim, Wags signs the Christmas card with her inked paw print. Underneath it says, 'Thanks for saving my life.' "

"That's nice."

"I didn't know Wags was sick. What did she have?"

"Nothing."

"I don't understand."

"I don't either but, as you said, Virginia Allen is an emotional woman."

Selling Magnets to Make Beer Money

HARDWARE disease was once a major problem of cattle. They have a rough tongue that has a propensity for pulling grass, grain, nails, baling wire, or anything they can grasp or lick into their mouths for swallowing. They never worry about the consistency of what they swallow. After all, they have four stomachs at the end of their esophagus to sort things out. Why waste time on that in the mouth cavity? The first stomach (the rumen or paunch) serves as a fermentation vat to break down the roughage they consume. The second stomach (the reticulum, along with its more conventional physiological function) serves as a depository for the hardware swallowed. The problem is that the reticulum is separated from the cardiac cavity containing the heart by only the diaphragm. The gravity of the area tends to cause sharp-pointed objects to work forward, puncturing the wall of the reticulum and the diaphragm and then entering the cardiac cavity. This can set up a pericardial infection and practically always causes death.

In my father's prime, nothing further was attempted after the diagnosis. During my practice days, attempts were being made to treat the problem if it was not too advanced. One of the most heroic methods was surgical intervention. I would, with the owner's consent, do a rumenotomy that would surgically expose the inside of the rumen through an incision in the upper left flank. The operation was done under local anesthesia with the cow confined, standing in a stanchion, or snubbed up in a corner of a box stall. There was little or no pain involved from the surgery. After draping the area to prevent leakage into the peritoneal cavity, I inserted a gloved hand and arm into the rumen, passed it on into the reticulum, and attempted to find the nail or piece of wire causing the problem. At times the objects were easily found and removed, and the cow would make a spectacular recovery. Other times the results would be less than desired. Either the object causing the problem could not be found or extensive peritoneal or pericardial infection had already occurred, negating any benefit to be derived from removing the offending piece of metal. The price I charged for the surgery was minimal—far less than for comparable surgery in St. Margaret's Hospital. No surgery would have been done there at comparable rates. Successful surgery was good advertisement. Unsuccessful surgery was never forgotten. However, the alternative was generally death, so I persisted in my efforts during those days.

Later, some advances were made. One advance was a metal detector to actually pinpoint the metal. As most cattle had metal in their stomachs, this had to be accompanied by clinical symptoms to be of value.

Still later, magnets became available for use. These were approximately two and one-half inches long by one-half inch in diameter. They were administered through the mouth by a balling gun—an instrument used to administer pills, capsules, and the like to large animals. A couple of magnets were often administered, hoping to magnetically clamp onto the metal and prevent penetration or further penetration of the metal. An instrument was made that could even be passed into the stomach. It had a magnet at the end and was supposed to be of value in retrieving metal or previously administered magnets from the reticulum. In hope or desperation, I used magnets promiscuously.

One evening, after leaving work, I stopped by Dutch Kelsey's meat-packing house. Dutch, a wiry built man with slightly humped shoulders, was just finishing up the day's chores. He was nearly always on the run and acquired the humped shoulders from the forward projection of the upper part of his body accelerating his constant movement. He invited me to have a beer with him. He kept a few cases in his cooler for just such situations. Never being one to turn down a free beer, I readily agreed. I had stopped to inquire about the progress for preparing the meat for the barbecue at the next county fair. Dutch assured me that all the meat had been prepared and was stored in boxes at the back of his cooler awaiting the day. The talk drifted on to other subjects as we started on the second beer.

"Doc, you know those magnets you're dosing these cattle with?"

"Sure, why?"

"Well, we butcher a lot of those cattle. We could recover those magnets, and you could use them over again."

"Yes, I suppose that is right."

At this juncture Tom, the butcher, entered the front room where we were seated on the counter finishing off our second beer. Tom wore an unbuttoned sleeveless denim shirt, trousers, and thongs. He was still drying off his arms with a towel.

"Tom, get a beer for yourself from the cooler and join us. Better make it three. You'll have another, won't you, Doc? Been a hot day out there."

"Sure, why not." I had already forgotten Marian's request to be home early as we had to go to the Jaycees' Award Dinner.

"Tom, how many animals did we kill today? I haven't got the count yet."

"Twenty head of cattle and ten of hogs," Tom answered. "I was knee deep in blood and guts for awhile."

"Doc, we're killing quite a few cattle these days. Just think if we recovered two magnets from each steer for reuse. What do you pay for these magnets?"

"They cost me one dollar each. I sell them for two dollars to the farmer or administer them myself for two-fifty."

"Look, Doc, suppose I sold these back to you for fifty cents each. I'd make fifty cents and you'd save fifty cents each. Nobody could tell if these magnets were used or not."

"Yes, I suppose that is right."

"Look, Doc, every bovine needs a couple of those magnets."

"Well, it couldn't hurt them, and it would help in a lot of cases to prevent trouble."

"All you need to do is sell the farmers on using them," Tom observed.

"Well, Tom, that's easier said than done."

"How much do those magnets weigh?" asked Dutch. "If they weigh enough, the farmer could recover the cost when he has his cattle weighed at sale. You know Horace, down at the sales barn, always sells his cattle on a water fill. Cheaper than hay, he says."

"Water is cheaper than magnets too."

"Maybe we could require that all cattle going back to the farm or feedlot be given magnets."

"That would take time to do."

"Not for you. You could get Swede, who helps Armer vaccinate the pigs, to do the work. Pay him two bits a magnet. You could sure make beer money without trouble."

"Even pretzel money too, huh?" I added. "Only one problem. It would have to be state law."

"No problem. We'll get Tom McVey to introduce the bill at the next legislative session in Topeka. If a person contributes one hundred dollars to his campaign fund, he'll introduce any bill. He always says he would outlaw mother-in-laws for a two hundred and fifty dollar contribution."

"Well one hundred dollars would be the money I'd save on two hundred magnets you recovered." I was beginning to run figures through my head. "Say, how's the beer holding out?"

"Tom, see if you can't find another round. Doc and I are about to become millionaires."

We were halfway through the next round, figuring number of cattle, cost of labor, cost of magnets, and net profits when Louise, Dutch's wife, entered.

"Doc, Marian is tracking you down. Seems you're emcee at the Jaycees' Award Dinner tonight. You'd better get moving."

"Oh, damn. I completely forgot." I shook my head to clear it and dashed out the door.

"Tom, that Award Dinner ought to be some affair tonight. Doc was getting in prime form. He'll probaby end up naming a Young Woman of the Year rather than a Young Man of the Year."

"He probably will. Ought to make headlines in the newspaper tomorrow."

"Yea, it'd be a first. Louise and I should have gone."

"Well, it's too late now. Need another beer? Louise isn't hollering at you yet."

"Sure, why not? Young Woman of the Year—that ought to be quite a night. Tom, seriously, we ought to be able to make money recovering those magnets. We could sell them to farmers if Doc wouldn't buy them."

"It would make beer money anyway, wouldn't it?"

Dr. Armer Up a Tree

PAT and Mike were riding with me in my station wagon as we made our way back from the western part of Fred Hunter's ranch. The screwworm season was upon the area and we had been out there treating a cow who had gotten scratched up and then blown by screwworm flies, which lay eggs on open wounds. As we passed back through one of the pastures, Pat pointed to a scrawny oak tree isolated over by a draw that bisected this particular pasture. Pat burst out laughing and elbowed his brother, Mike.

"Remember the time that cow had Dr. Armer treed up that tree, Mike?"

"I sure do. I never knew a cripple like Dr. Armer could climb so fast," Mike said as he joined in the laughter.

My ears pricked up. This was obviously a story I hadn't previously heard. "Armer, treed?" I asked. "This I haven't heard. Fill me in on the details."

Pat and Mike both continued laughing for a few minutes. Finally Pat calmed down sufficiently to start the story. "Well, it was last summer. The day was a scorcher, just like today. You were out someplace so Fred told us to get Armer to come out. We had a cow down under the tree so Fred decided to invest the money in having a veterinarian look at her."

"She'd been sick for a couple of days. You know, moving slow, not staying up with the herd," Mike explained. "When she got clear down, Fred decided it was time to call. He wasn't about to waste money paying a veterinarian for a cow still on her feet."

"Of course not," I added.

"Anyway, Armer followed us on out here in his car. We were in the pickup in front of him to show him the way to drive. Offered to take him in the pickup, but he said he needed the medicine in his car," Pat explained.

"Well, you got out here. Then what happened?" I asked.

"Armer went down and looked at the cow real seriouslike. He took her temperature, lifted up her eyelids, and looked at the membranes—all that veterinary stuff. Finally, he said that she probably had that anaplasmosis," said Pat.

"That's too big a word, Pat. I think he called it yellow fever. You're just showing off with that 'osis' word."

"Aw now, Mike, let me tell Doc this story. He wants to hear about Armer getting treed. He doesn't care whether the cow had anaplasmosis, yellow fever, pneumonia, or whatever."

"O.K. Just trying to help explain," apologized Mike.

"Anyway, Armer went back up to his car and got a syringe full of medicine. He brought the syringe and a nose lead back down the slope to where the cow was lying under the tree. It was hot and she had probably picked that spot for the little shade it offered," continued Pat.

"Armer told me to get that nose lead in the cow's nose and pull her head around to the side tight," interjected Mike. "He jabbed a needle into her jugular vein and shot that syringe of medicine into that vein."

Pat cut in. "If I'm ever that far down I want Armer to shoot the same medicine into me. He had no sooner pulled the needle out than that cow was on her feet and spitting mad."

"Yes, she was," agreed Mike. "She shook that nose lead out of her nose, lowered her head, snorted a couple of times, and charged towards Armer."

Pat continued the story. I stopped the car so I could follow the story as they described it. "Armer was too far from his car or our pickup to make a run for either even if he hadn't been crippled. He saw that tree behind him. There was no place else to go. Mike and I were hauling on the cow's tail but she wasn't paying any attention to us. Armer swatted the cow's head a couple of times with his cane, just enough to detract her. In those few moments he turned and climbed up that little scrub oak faster than greased lightning. The cow charged and hit the tree as Armer was getting up out of reach. There was Armer up above swinging a cane at the cow every time she looked at him. It was hilarious. She couldn't get him, and he couldn't get down."

"But it became damned serious within a few minutes," added Mike. "The cow looked around at us hanging on her tail, decided we might be easier to reach than Armer, and turned and charged."

"Talk about bowlegged cowboys running. We ran for that pickup fast as our legs would carry us with that cow snorting at our heels. I was ahead so I had time to dash around to the other side and get the cab door opened and climb inside. Mike, here, wasn't that fast. He just dived and rolled under the truck as the cow's head hit the side. That whole truck started raising up on its side. I thought the cow was going to go under the pickup with Mike."

Mike continued the story. "The cow backed off and the pickup settled down on four wheels again. I didn't waste any time. I scooted out from under that truck on the other side, opened the door by Pat, and climbed over him to the other side nearest the cow. By that time the cow was sizing things up. She'd look first at the truck and then down the slope at Armer perched up in that tree. She decided she'd try the truck again. She saw me sitting there gawking out the window at her and charged. I got the glass rolled up just as she arrived. Somehow or the other she didn't break the glass, but there she was on the other side of that glass snorting and ranting. I yelled at Pat to get the pickup started and get out of there."

"We got away from that cow fast, and I mean fast. Armer was still down below though so when we got to the top of the slope, we stopped and looked back. We couldn't leave him stranded." Pat was describing what happened next. "The cow decided to go after Armer again. She charged that oak tree and was butting away at its trunk and shaking the hell out of the tree, while Armer was hunched down in a fork just out of reach and trying to use his cane to knock that cow down. He would have needed a two-by-four to have made an impression on her. I told Mike to get back in the pickup bed and get his rope ready. As I drove by he could lay the loop over her head and we could drag her away from Armer and that tree."

Mike took over the story. "Pat told me that all right. He was driving, so he wasn't worried. I told him there was no place to snub the cow to except the tree that Armer was in or the trailer hitch behind the pickup. Armer wasn't going to be able to get down out of the tree with the cow tied below, and I was too scared to get down on the ground and try to snub that cow to the trailer hitch. Anyway, Pat convinced me to get in back and we would drive by the cow. He assured me that I ought to be able to attract the cow away from the tree and Armer. He was certainly right." Mike, followed by Pat, burst out laughing again.

When they had gotten over the outburst, I asked them to continue. "Dad has never told me about this. I'm still listening."

"Well, the idea worked even better than Pat had imagined. Pat drove the pickup down in back of the cow. I reached out and gave the cow a few good swats with my curled up lariat. Man, did that get her mad. She started to turn around, Pat was gunning the motor to be ready to make tracks, and the next thing I knew the cow was climbing in that pickup bed with me. Pat was gunning her like hell to get up this here slope. I was scared half out of my wits with that cow coming in after me. I managed to get over the top of that cab and onto the hood of the motor before that cow any more than got a sniff of me. That didn't stop her but just a few seconds though. Then she started over the cab top after me. I jumped off and fast. I was scared. Somehow she got herself straddled over the top of that cab and didn't come after me."

It was Pat's turn to continue the story. "It would have been funny as all get out if I hadn't been so scared. There was Mike coming over the top of the cab and landing in front of me on the hood. In a few moments the cow's front feet appeared down in front of the windshield and Mike rolled off the other side and scampered like hell towards Armer's car, which was just a short distance away. I didn't know what was going to happen for a few minutes. The cow kept jumping with her hindlegs trying to propel herself on over. I didn't want any part of that so I swerved sharp to see if I could roll her off. Somehow I succeeded. However, when she was about ready to roll off, she managed to get back on her rear legs and made a jump out of the truck bed, landing cleanly on all four feet. It was beautiful."

"Beautiful, my foot. I jumped in Armer's car and got it started. Luckily the cow was completely winded by now and just stood there weaving on her legs and panting like she was ready to take her last breath. I drove down by the tree and hollered at Armer. He practically fell out of that tree, he was so eager to get away. He grabbed the nose lead and syringe off the ground, jumped into the passenger seat, and yelled at me to get out of there. Anyway, we all got away before the cow regained her wind."

"What happened to the cow?"

"Oh, she died. They all do. Fred doesn't call a vet until they are practically dead."

"Some of those prolapse uterus cases I replace live, don't they?"

"Yea, that's right. You've got a pretty good record sticking those calfbeds back inside. Fred lets us call you on the first day on those. He knows they will die if not put back in. Not those other cases, though. He wants to wait and see if they'll get better by themselves."

"The trouble with Fred's cattle is that they're wild. Take that cow you were talking about. She had anaplasmosis which means she was anemic. If she had been calm, she might have lived. But, being wild, she killed herself because she didn't have enough red blood cells to provide oxygen for all that exertion."

"You're right on that but these are wild cattle. We can't get those wild bulls up out of the pastures so they're never culled. As Sean O'Dell, the Irishman who used to work for Fred says, 'Fred's got great-grandfathers breeding their own great-granddaughters. That's what you call incest, I guess, but worse yet, Fred's deliberately line breeding for wildness. Those wild bulls are there doing the breeding until they drop over from old age.' Fred won't let us shoot them, and there isn't a cow pony around that can turn them when they break back at roundup time."

I dropped the brothers off at the ranch house. Fred was away. They said he'd be by to pay me someday.

The next Sunday I brought the event up with my father. I could tell immediately that he was displeased. "If Mike had held on to the nose lead, it would never have happened. Fred should still have Sean O'Dell working for him."

"But Sean went to work at the cement plant. Makes more there in an hour than he did in an entire day working for Fred. Sean has a family to support."

"Stockmen can't pay those kind of wages," argued my father. "Labor unions are going to ruin this country."

I saw this argument wasn't getting anyplace so I said, "Pat says if he ever gets real sick he wants you to give him some of that medicine."

My father started smiling. "I'll be glad to. I just want Sean O'Dell to hold that nose lead in Pat's nose. He won't let him get loose."

Desexing Mrs. Bradshaw's Immoral Dogs

"DR. Porter, this is Sarah Bradshaw calling."

"Yes, Mrs. Bradshaw. What can I do for you?"

"You can fix my male dogs."

"Of course. When can you bring them in?"

Mrs. Bradshaw lived out west of Buxton on the Wilson-Elk county line. She was a widow who had lost her husband some years back. Now she lived alone on her farm and rented out the land.

"Dr. Porter, there's nine of them. I can't bring them in. You'll have to come out."

"You said fix them, didn't you? I presume you mean castrate."

"Yes, that's the word. I've got to get them fixed."

"I don't think I can do that out there. I'll need them at my office Mrs. Bradshaw—you did say nine? That's a lot of dogs to castrate."

"I know. I know. But those males are acting horrible. Betty, one of my females, is in season and they won't leave her alone if I let her out of her room."

"Well, that is bothersome, but why don't you have her spayed?"

"Spayed? You mean desexed? Dr. Porter, I can tell you aren't a woman. How would you like to have your internal organs removed? That's just horrible."

"Now, Mrs. Bradshaw. That may be right, but to castrate nine dogs rather than spay one female doesn't seem equitable."

"There you go again. Is that right to take the sex organs out of a female? Besides I have three female dogs, not just one."

"I see. But it is going to be hard to restrain the dogs for anesthesia at your farm. I need them at my office."

"Dr. Porter, I can't do that. There's nine of them."

"Mrs. Bradshaw, you can bring them in one or two at a time, can't you?"

"Of course not. Dr. Porter, these males aren't able to control their passions. It's terrible. I won't stand for it another day. You get out here tomorrow or I'll have to call your father."

I was pushed into a corner. I had no alternative. "All right, Mrs. Bradshaw. Tomorrow afternoon at 2:00 P.M. O.K.?"

"The sooner the better."

After I hung up I pondered on my problem. Clarence was away at that time but I might be able to get Swede, the man who helped my father at the sales barn, to go with me. I could take a collapsible table to use for surgery. The matter of anesthesia still bothered me. We didn't have the choice of anesthetics we now have. While considering this problem, I remembered an article that I had read recently in the *Journal*. The writer wrote of using pentobarbital intramuscularly with excellent results. Intramuscular injection would be a snap. Mrs. Bradshaw and I could handle that without assistance. I relaxed and looked forward to the next day's experience. Why hadn't someone told me about intramuscular injection of pentobarbital years ago?

The next afternoon I drove up the tree-shaded lane to Sarah Bradshaw's house. It was a large, two-storied, white-painted frame house with a wide porch extending the entire width of the front. A porch swing was suspended on one side of the porch and two cane chairs and a settee were on the other side. A set of wide steps led from the porch down to a sidewalk that ran down to the circular drive that curved in front of the house.

Mrs. Bradshaw stood at the top of the steps awaiting my arrival. She was a slim lady of medium height with sharp facial features. She was dressed in a checkered dress with a waist belt pulled tight to accent her slim figure. On her head she wore a bonnet made of the same checkered material as her dress. Her entire appearance bespoke a spinster lady who had a no-nonsense approach towards life.

"Dr. Porter, I'm sure glad you came. I don't think I could put up with those male dogs of mine another day. I love them all but they can't control their base instincts."

"Mrs. Bradshaw, I can take that instinct out of one end but I can't necessarily take it out of the head at the other end."

"Oh, you will, Dr. Porter. I was married. I know all about those male instincts. This country would be better off if half the men were desexed."

"But who would do the picking of the half to undergo the surgery?"

"They could start in on all those criminals in our prisons. There were times I thought my husband, Jacob, should have been desexed. We didn't have any children. He seemed to be concerned only with passion."

"I certainly hope you don't think I should be castrated?"

"Dr. Porter, I didn't bring you out here to talk about that. The dogs are penned up on the back porch. Drive around to the back of the house."

I drove around to the back, got out my syringes and pentobarbital, and explained to Sarah Bradshaw what I was going to do.

Mrs. Bradshaw did indeed have the nine male dogs, cocker spaniels of assorted colors, penned up on her back porch.

"Dr. Porter, I will carry them out one at a time and you can inject them. How long will it keep them anesthetized?"

"An hour or more. Let's inject all of them and then start the surgery. The surgery shouldn't take long."

Sarah Bradshaw carried out each dog. I injected it and she released it.

"They won't run off," she assured me.

I injected all nine dogs and then set up my surgery table and instrument stand. When I was ready, I looked around for the first patient. To my consternation, only two of the dogs were apparently anesthetized. The others were staggering around and falling over each other.

Well, maybe they just needed more time. With Sarah Bradshaw's assistance, I rapidly did the requested surgical procedures on the two anesthetized dogs.

The other seven dogs were still staggering around. I was in a quandry. I had gone too far. I couldn't change methods of anesthesia now. Besides, Sarah Bradshaw wasn't going to be of any help in restraint for intravenous anesthesia—even if I could have calculated the amount to use safely on top of the intramuscular injection.

I had to run a bluff with Sarah Bradshaw. I couldn't plead incompetence in the procedure I used. There was no need to wait longer.

"Mrs. Bradshaw, this occurs sometimes. We'll just supplement it with a local anesthesia and proceed."

"Dr. Porter, you don't need to take all the pain away. They have had some very evil ideas in their minds and shouldn't get off too easy."

The error in handling the method of anesthesia didn't backfire as I feared. Sarah Bradshaw was irritated with the morals of her male dogs and she took some pleasure in seeing them castrated even if they were partly conscious.

"Serves them right. They won't leave poor Betty alone."

As I drove away from her place that afternoon, after she gave me her thanks for my professional services in helping her out of an unpleasant situation, I thought I had come out of the situation "smelling like a rose." I'd never use that method of anesthesia again. Better still, I'd write to the editor of the *Journal* that night giving him an earful for letting an article promoting that type of anesthesia get into print.

How to Make a Million Dollars

JIM, this is Sally," said the voice on the telephone.

"Sally who?"

"Sally Harris, John's wife. Don't you recognize my voice?"

"Of course. Now I do. Sally, I'm sorry. I don't get calls from you very often. To what do I owe the honor of this call?"

"Jim, John is real sick this week. Kidney stones, the doctor says. He can hardly move because of the pain."

"Sally, I'm sorry. I do hope he gets to feeling better."

"I'm sure he will but he needs help now."

"Well, I hope he gets it."

"Jim, you don't understand. He needs a veterinarian to run the practice until he gets back on his feet. You have a veterinarian working for you, don't you?"

"Yes, why do you ask?"

"Send him over here. John needs help."

"I can't do that. Dr. Smart has a wife and children here. His wife wouldn't want him running off."

"It's only for a few days. You can surely send him up for that length of time to help out your old buddy."

"Now don't start calling him old. I'm the same age as he is. Sally, I'll tell you what I'll do for John. I'll come up myself. This is Saturday night. John can beg off on Sunday calls. I'll be there tomorrow evening and spend the week. I presume you'll provide bed and board?"

"Of course. Come over tomorrow afternoon. We'll have supper together and, if there are any calls that can't be postponed until Monday, you can take care of them tomorrow night."

"Be damned sure they can't be postponed or I won't come up until tomorrow night."

"Jim, you come up tomorrow afternoon or John will get out of his sick bed to answer those calls. He wants to take care of everything in the county. Does more than the other three veterinarians in the county combined."

"Sally, I still don't understand. Three other veterinarians in the county and he has to call an outsider in to help?"

"Jim, John is afraid to let another veterinarian get on a client's farm. Afraid he would lose that client. Says it's far easier to keep clients than to get new ones."

"I suppose that's right. I was never in that situation. Well, I'll be over tomorrow afternoon. Tell John I'm certain that he won't get run out of practice by those competitors."

"I'll tell him but he runs scared. I'll have supper ready by six. John will give you time to eat before you start working."

"If he doesn't, I'll drive back home tomorrow night."

I drove into Harris's driveway the next afternoon shortly before six and was met at the door by Sally.

"Jim, come on in. Supper will be on the table in a few minutes."

I entered and shut the door behind me. After a quick glance around the room, "Nice place you have here, Sally."

"Glad you like it, Jim. Now you can freshen up in the bathroom, first door to the left down that hall, and then say hello to John in his bedroom, second door to the right. I'll have supper on the table by the time you get back. John is taking calls on the telephone at his bedside. He'll bring you up to date."

"No wonder he's sick. Never gets away from the telephone."

"Do you? You vets are all alike, aren't you?" She grinned and hurried out a door opposite the direction she had previously indicated as leading to the bathroom and John's bedroom.

A few minutes later I peeked into John's bedroom. He was lying on his side, legs drawn up, and eyes closed. I slipped in and instantly one eye opened. "Jim, it's time you got here. Knew you wouldn't let a buddy down. Come over and sit down."

I walked over and stood looking down at John. "John, I'm sure sorry you're laid up. Sally says you have kidney stones."

"The doctor says that, not Sally. She wouldn't know kidney stones from heart worms. Did you every have stones, Jim?"

"Can't say that I have, John."

"Don't ever get them, Jim. They are the most painful thing that can happen to a person. Even worse than having a baby."

"How do you know? Had a baby?"

"Of course not, Jim. But it's worse. Nothing could be more painful than these stones. They have to pass through those little ureters to get out and the ureters won't dilate." He grabbed at his side and stopped speaking for a few minutes. Sweat drops started popping out on his forehead.

"Got a pain, John?"

"Yes, one of those spasms. God, they're excruciating. Jim, get me one of those pink pills over there." I handed it to him and he popped it into his mouth. "Now pass that glass of water over here. Put the straw in my mouth." He took a few sips, said nothing for several minutes, and then slowly began to relax and straighten his legs out.

"See all those pills there on the bed stand?"

"Yes, you do have a collection."

"I do, don't I? Well I've learned more materia medica since these stones started bothering me this last year than I ever did at college. If we get time, I'll give you an education."

"Thanks but I hope I never have to be treated for stones."

"Jim, I hope so too. It's excruciating."

"John, to get down to business, is there anything I need to do tonight?"

"I'm sure there is. I've been writing down notes as the telephone calls come in. Here, let me read my note pad." He picked up a tablet from the bed stand and studied it for a few minutes. "Jim, most of these calls can be postponed until tomorrow. I'll go easy on you. If I was doing it, I'd go tonight, but since you're new here, you can handle them tomorrow. Here is one call you'd better answer tonight though."

"Tell me about it?"

"It's Jack Parker who lives out north of town. He has a sick cow. He's real difficult to please. If I don't get you out there tonight, he's liable to call one of those other veterinarians."

"I'd think you would like to lose those difficult characters to the other vets."

"Jim, I don't like to lose any large-animal clients to them. Let them split up the doggy and kitty business here in town. I want the cow and pig work. That's where the money is."

"What are you going to do with all this money, John?"

"Probably build a bigger house for Sally. How do you like this house, Jim?"

"It's real elegant, John."

"I hope so. It cost me $75,000 to put up. All paid for, too."

"It's nice to be able to afford to do that."

"Jim, I'll teach you how to make money this week and you also can build big houses. Have you made your first million yet?"

"I doubt it. At least I haven't saved it."

"I thought so. I'm about ready to start on my third million."

"That's good to hear, but I hope you don't kill yourself earning it. Do you ever get any rest except when you're sick like now?"

"Of course. I probably average four or five hours sleep a night. That's all a person needs."

"That may be so, but I sure like to get more when I can."

"Jim, you aren't a newlywed anymore. Five hours sleep is plenty, but we're wasting time. Got work to do. Sally will probably have supper on the table—you still call it supper, don't you?" I nodded. "Well, get out there and eat a bite. Afterwards I'll tell you how to get out to Parker's farm." As I was going out his bedroom door he called after me. "Don't take too long eating. Parker won't want to wait."

Sally did have supper on the table. She introduced me to David, their ten-year-old boy and only child, and the three of us sat down to eat.

"Sally, I sometimes put in long hours but it's because I have to. I think John enjoys working these hours."

"I'm not certain about that and I live with him. It may be the money. If he knew how to make as much money as a stockbroker, he might be just as happy."

"It would sure be a lot easier," I commented.

"Well, you and John studied to be vets. That's how he knows to make money, so he's out to see how many millions he can make as a vet."

"I'd think you two have enough salted away so you could retire and live on your investments."

"Probably so, but John wouldn't be happy. If there is another dollar to be made out there doctoring cows, he wants to make it."

"I'm glad I don't practice in the same county with John. He'd run me out of business."

"He probably would," agreed Sally.

When I had finished cleaning up my plate, Sally suggested that I have my dessert and coffee when I returned from the evening's work. If I delayed longer now, John would just be nervous. I excused myself and returned to John's bedroom.

"Thought you'd never get through, Jim. What are you trying to do, get fat?"

I ignored the question. "O.K., John, where does this Jack Parker live?"

John gave me directions. I was to drive his practice car. Anything I needed would be in the trunk. When I inquired about charges, he told me not to worry. Howard, his office man, took care of collections. That way John didn't have to lose time making collections.

"That sounds good, John. I wish I had an office person capable of doing that. If I didn't get my pay as I went, at least wherever possible, I would probably have to close the doors."

"Jim, you need a Howard. Look for one. It'll sure cut down on wasted time and give you more time to make calls. Pay attention to me this week while you're here and you too can make a million dollars."

"O.K. Get some rest. I'll take care of Parker."

"I know you will, Jim. Sure glad you came over." Saying this, he stretched out and closed his eyes.

I went back to the dining room, got the car keys from Sally, and drove out to Parker's. Jack Parker was expecting my arrival. He came out to meet and direct me to the barn.

"Dr. Harris said he was sending another person out. Said he was sick. Is it serious?"

"Anytime Dr. Harris can't make it, it's serious. He's a dedicated veterinarian. Apparently he has kidney stones."

"I sure hope he gets all right. He's a real good vet when he slows down. Would sure hate to lose him."

"I don't think you'll lose him. Where's the sick cow?"

"In the barn. Been off feed and not chewing her cud since morning. Come on in and take a look."

He flipped on the lights inside the barn door and led me back to look at a cow confined in a stanchion. An examination revealed nothing too serious bothering the cow. Evidently indigestion from something she ate. As I was making the examination and treating the cow, Jack Parker continued talking. After he gave me the clinical history and the life history on the cow, he got back to talking about Dr. Harris.

"Yes, sir. Dr. Harris would be an excellent veterinarian if he'd just slow down. When he drives into the yard, he's always in a hurry. Has the cow treated before I even give him the history. Some day he is going to run into trouble doing that. May end up treating a cow for pneumonia that's having calving trouble."

"Well, I hardly think that will happen, Dr. Harris does stay on the run though."

After an appropriate time, I excused myself and returned to the Harrises. Sally met me as I came in.

"Take care of things O.K., I presume?"

"No fatalities."

"Good. Get your bag from your car and get unpacked. Use the first bedroom down the hall on the right. I'll get some apple pie for you. You didn't get your dessert for supper. What do you want to drink? I do have some decaffeinated coffee. Won't keep you awake."

"That'll be fine."

After I brought my bag in, I rejoined Sally at the table for the pie and coffee. "I presume you see more of John now since he is laid up than usual?"

"I suppose but it's hardly any pleasure with his moaning and groaning. Jim, you need to sleep fast. I'll have breakfast on the table about 6:15 A.M. John's asleep now so I won't bother him. He'll be awake and ready to give orders then, though. By the way, what do you want for breakfast—bacon with eggs over lightly O.K.?"

"Sounds fine."

"Wanted to be sure. You'll have a long day ahead. No telling when you'll eat next."

The next morning I found John at the breakfast table when I came into the room.

"How do you feel, John?"

"Horrible, Jim, but I'll live. How did you make out with Parker?" he asked.

"Fine. He thinks you're a good vet."

"He doesn't act like it. Always talking about those other vets."

"John, he thinks you're in too big a hurry."

"Hurry, hell, he wants to spend an hour telling about the flu he had last winter. I'd starve to death if I had to wait for him to get through talking."

"I don't think so, but what's up for today? I presume the telephone is still ringing."

"Yes, I've got you lined up. Sure hope you can handle it, Jim."

"I came over here to do that. Just relax, John."

"Jim, can you handle twenty-six farm calls in a day?"

"Well, I never have, but I'll sure try."

"Don't expect you to. Just asked. That's my record. Twenty-six calls in one day. I think that's a Kansas record. The state vet association ought to give me a plaque. You can't spend time visiting with people like Jack Parker and do that."

"I guess not."

Sally appeared with a platter of bacon and eggs and set them before us. "You eating, John?" she asked.

"Just juice and coffee, Sally. Trying to flush those stones through."

"Jim, pitch in. I'll get you both some juice and coffee. The toast will be ready in a few minutes. Need anything else?"

"No, Sally, that ought to take care of me."

"Jim, while you're eating, I'll fill you in. The first stop will be out at the Ivan Schultz dairy south of town. He'll have his dairy herd up for testing. He'll have all the paper work ready—tag numbers, ages, breeds, and the like. You just get the bloods and do the TB testing. Take the paperwork in to Howard. He'll handle that part. You can go back Thursday and read the tuberculin tests. Understand?"

"Sure, no problem." I was enjoying a leisurely breakfast while John was rifling through his notes.

"Now, Jim, you haven't got all day. We'll feed you but don't play with your food. Time is money and the calls are waiting. When you get through at the Schultzes, go back to my office. Howard will be there by then, and he and I will have gotten your morning's work lined up."

"John, Sally would be unhappy if I ate any faster. She'd think I didn't enjoy her cooking."

"Don't be so sure of that."

He gave me directions to Ivan Schultz's and to his office. "Now, Jim, don't drive like a sightseer. I know we have beautiful scenery around here but you're here to work. That car was built to go over one hundred miles per hour. Don't waste time on the roads. Remember, twenty-six calls a day is the record. You don't want to look bad."

"John, you haven't told Jim about some of those near misses you've had. The time you were coming over the top of the hill at eighty-five miles per hour and a wheel bearing froze in your rear wheel. He'd better not try to emulate you at that speed. He might not be as lucky as you've been."

"Jim, I guess Sally is right. But don't poke around or I'll have to put you on a piece-work commission."

I smiled, excused myself, and drove out to the Schultzes. Ivan and his wife, Maria, came out to meet me. Maria had the paperwork ready. After introductions we went back to the barn and into the milking parlor where one string of cows was confined in their stanchions. The health records that had to be filled out called for TB and blood tests and physical examinations of the udders, so we proceeded.

While we were working, the conversation revealed that the Schultzes, Mennonites, had relatives in the Fredonia area who were my clients. During the Dust Bowl years of the thirties, most of the

Mennonites in western Kansas had been blown out. The Okies, under similar circumstances, headed for California on Highway 66. The Mennonites moved east in Kansas. Part of them, like the Schultzes, had settled in this area, and the others had moved into Wilson County and were now my clients. Naturally they had many relatives and acquaintances in the Wilson County group, so we had much to converse about.

When I finished with the work, I returned to the office and introduced myself to Howard. "Dr. Porter, you're running about thirty minutes behind Dr. Harris's schedule, and he's real nervous. Wants you to call him to get the next list of calls. After you get through talking with him, I'll fill you in on directions."

"O.K. What's the telephone number at home?"

"Same as here. I'll ring for you."

A few moments later I was talking to John. "What's holding you up, Jim? You're behind schedule now."

"Well, I did have to make a physical exam of those udders. I don't have to do that for the milk companies in my areas."

"Jim, that shouldn't take any time. What are you, a sex deviate and playing with those teats? You've got to move faster or you won't get done today."

"Well, I'll try. Incidentally these Mennonites you work for are related to the Mennonites in my county."

"Fine, you can come up here for one of their church get-togethers. You can stay at my house and spend the day eating and visiting with them, but you've got to work today."

"Yes, John," I smiled to myself. This week promised to be interesting.

John gave me instructions on a list of clients to see in the southwest part of the county. I should be able to get back to the office in the early afternoon, he assured me, and then he would give me my next itinerary. After he hung up, I got directions from Howard and started out. Some twelve calls later and at about 7:00 P.M., I drove into the Harris's driveway.

Sally answered the doorbell and admitted me. "Freshen up and I'll get your supper on the table."

"How's John feeling?"

"Got some rest today. Dr. Wilkerson did stop by. He says John is going to come through it without surgery. Prescribed another medicine. John is going to be a real junkie by the time this is over."

I excused myself to clean up. A short time later I was eating supper with Sally. David had eaten earlier. "John will be joining us in a few minutes," Sally informed me. "He's worried about anybody else's ability to run his practice so wants to talk to you. Give him a good report. I'd like to get him out of here when he gets better and go on a long trip to Hawaii."

"I'll do my best to reassure him."

At this time John entered the room and joined us at the table. "Jim, was it too much for you today?"

"No, I'm fresh as a daisy and ready to go. How many more calls?"

"Only three. You should be in bed by 11:00 P.M. A real slow day. I wonder if they know I'm sick and are calling those other vets. Jim, you've got to make a good impression. Can't afford to lose a client."

"John, I think I'm holding it together for you. The clients all expressed their sorrow on your illness and hoped you'd get better."

"Jim, people are like that. They say one thing out of one side of their mouth and telephone the competing vet out of the other side."

"John, your practice will survive your illness. Just follow the doctor's orders and get better."

Just then the telephone rang. Sally answered it. "It's for you, John. Here, I'll carry the phone to the table. Just sit where you are."

John took the phone from her hand. "Hello, Dr. Harris here." (A pause.) "Well, I'm happy to hear that, but I'd be glad to send Dr. Porter if you had any doubts." (Another pause.) "All right, I'm sorry Dr. Porter couldn't get there earlier today. He's new here, you know." (Another pause.) "No, I'm going to live. Thank you. Good night."

He put the phone back on its base and turned to me. "Jim, I just lost five dollars. That would have been a fifteen dollar call if you could have made it today after he first called. The cow has gotten well and so you won't have to go tonight. Only two calls for tonight. Jim, that's the reason for the speed. You need to get there before the cow dies or gets well. It's real hard to charge if the animal isn't sick. Now here is an example and I lose five dollars."

"I think you'll survive, John," Sally interjected. "Let Jim eat his supper in peace before you send him out again."

"Jim, I'm sorry. Eat in peace. Say, how's Marian? I haven't seen her in years."

"She's just fine, John. Sent her condolences on your illness."

"Thank her for me. How many children have you got now?"

"Three. Two girls and a boy. Slow on getting started but have got a family now."

"That's real nice, Jim. We only have one. I don't have time to take care of the home front now. Too busy."

"You can say that again," Sally added.

"Well, David seems to be quite a boy. Takes after you, doesn't he, John?" I thought it best to change the subject.

After some discussion about David, John returned to a summary of the day's activities. "Have any troubles today, Jim?"

"Not that I know of, John."

"Well you only handled twelve calls between 7:00 A.M. and 7:00 P.M. and only two left for this evening. That's only fourteen calls. What took so long?"

"I thought that was real good, John. I'd like to have that many calls on an average and an office man like Howard to handle the collections."

"Howard's real good, isn't he? Needs two weeks off a year to handle his wheat crop and doesn't have anything else to do the rest of the time so helps me to keep out of mischief. Good man, Howard."

"He is."

"Jim, is there any advice I can give you to speed up things? For instance, you had two cleaning jobs to do [cleaning refers to removing placentas that are not shed normally from the cow's uterus after the calf birth], how long did they take?"

"About thirty minutes each place. They were stuck tight to those buttons."

"Thirty minutes! Jim, you never want to spend more than five minutes on one of those jobs. They're the real money-maker. If they aren't loose, just put a couple of those uterine boluses in the uterus, give her a shot of stilbesterol and penicillin and get the hell out of there. They'll do just as well as if you play inside of them with your fingers for another twenty-five minutes. What have you got, Jim, a sexual hang-up and like to play inside those cow's sex organs?"

"John, you tell me how you want it done here. This is your practice, so I'll do it your way."

"Jim, excuse me. I've been sick." We then went over the events of the day and the two calls remaining. After a second cup of coffee, I excused myself. Sally let me out the door, assuring me she'd whip up something for dessert before I got back. "Sure glad you came over, Jim. John needed that rest. Don't pay any attention to what he said this evening. Actually he's feeling better or he wouldn't have been complaining so much."

I smiled and left to finish up the day's work.

The next morning John was sitting at the table when I entered. He held an unlit cigar in one hand and a cup of coffee in the other. "You are feeling better I see. Got your stogie out."

"I sure am. Just like Dr. Wilkerson said, I'm getting better. He says I've got to stay home the rest of the week but he didn't say I had to lay off the cigars. Where's your cigar, Jim? You still smoke, don't you?"

"Too much, I'm afraid. I keep a box with me in the car. Didn't want to smoke in your house."

"I don't smoke much, Jim, I chew. Here, take a cigar for your eye-opener." He handed one to me he was carrying in the pocket of his bathrobe.

"Thanks, John. I'll light up after I get on the road."

"Here's food for you, Jim," Sally said as she placed a platter of pancakes and bacon before me. "You probably won't get a chance to eat again until night so better shovel it in. You eating, John?"

"No. Just drinking. Nothing alcoholic, mind you. Just trying to get this sand washed through me. Bring me a big glass of orange juice to go with the cup of coffee."

"O.K. How are you going to handle that? You've got a cigar in one hand and a cup of coffee in the other. I don't see a third hand."

"Sally, it's simple. I put the cup down and pick up the glass."

"That's what I thought. You never put the cigar down when you're healthy except when you're in bed or the bathtub."

"That's right, and I think I've got a method worked out to handle the cigar when I'm in the bathtub. It won't work in the shower, but I think it'll work in the bathtub."

"This you'll have to tell me about."

"Not now. We have a day's work to plan."

"O.K. Start plotting out the strategy. How much do you want to gross today?"

"Jim, don't be coarse. I do have a couple of more dairy herds to take care of this morning. That means you can go back and read the tuberculin tests in three days on Friday."

"Fine, what else?"

"Well, a call came in at 5:00 A.M. Didn't wake you up but it's a prolapsed calfbed. I presume cows throw their calfbeds down in Wilson County too?"

"Once in awhile."

"You do know how to replace them, right?"

"I think so."

"Fine. But don't waste time. Use plenty of postpituitary on them. They'll practically crawl back inside. We just don't have time for you to play with those sex organs, Jim. You've got to get over those sex hang-ups if you're to make that million dollars."

"We do use that drug in my part of the state too, John."

"Glad to hear it. I thought you might be real out of date down there in Wilson County. Wasn't right sure why they called your area the Balkans."

"That's just because we are located in the southeast part of Kansas and are contrary."

"You're contrary all right. Anyway, when you get the prolapse replaced and the two dairies taken care of, go to the office and Howard and I will have your schedule worked out for you."

"It looks like I'm going to be busy, so I'll forego that third stack of hotcakes and get started."

"You'd better, Jim. You'll get too fat. I'll provide you board, but I'll be damned if I'm going to provide more than a maintenance diet. Nothing in our contract says you're to get a fattening diet."

"That's right, John. Now give me directions."

After receiving directions and a last minute pep talk from John, Sally escorted me to the door.

"I think John has decided to live. He was up hunting for his box of cigars this morning."

"He does act livelier, doesn't he?"

I returned to the house about 7:30 P.M. and some thirteen calls later. John was stretched out on the couch watching television.

"Jim, do you ever watch this television?"

"Well, once in awhile when I have time. Why do you ask?"

"Jim, I've seen something on that thing today that I didn't think they would put on the air."

"You did. What was that?"

"Sally says it's called soap operas."

"I've heard about them but never have had time to watch them. What did you see?"

"Jim, it's immoral what they have on the picture tube. One woman was trying to steal another woman's husband in one program. In another, a man was trying to get in bed with another man's wife. There were a lot of other things along that line in one program after another. It was really shocking. I just don't know how people can stand watching that. I'll be happy when I can get back to work."

"I'm sure you will. How do you feel tonight?"

"Some better. How did you do today? Handle that prolapse O.K.?"

"I think so. Don't think you lost any clients today."

"I sure hope you're right. Good clients are hard to replace."

"Still chewing the same cigar you had this morning?"

"Heavens, no. That thing was a soggy mess by noon. Threw it away and started in on this one."

"It's about gone too."

"It is, isn't it? Jim, I think I'll start leaving the cellophane on the outside. They'll last longer that way."

"You could buy cheaper cigars. Then you could afford to chew tobacco rather than cellophane."

"I suppose that's right, but it would be degrading for a man in my position to buy anything cheaper than a twenty-five cent cigar. Imagine me with a White Owl cigar."

"That would be degrading for you, I suppose. But poor vets like me have to have cheap habits."

"Jim, you pay attention to the way I run this practice and you'll be chewing Dutch Masters."

"Well, I'm all ears as long as it doesn't lead to ulcers or kidney stones."

By this time Sally had my supper on the table. "Jim, come eat a bite. John and you can discuss cigars while you're eating."

"Jim, there's only one call for you this evening so take your time eating. I postponed the other calls until morning. Won't have you testing dairy cows tomorrow as that is Wednesday and you would have to read tuberculin tests on Saturday. That way you can take sick animal calls tomorrow morning and get out of here by the middle of the day on Saturday."

"You're all heart, John. Can you really afford to do that?"

"Probably not but, as you say, I'm all heart."

After eating, I excused myself and went out to take care of the evening call. It was a dairy cow suffering from acetonemia, a metabolic disease that sometimes accompanies calving. While treating the cow, Hiram Levinsky, the owner, was telling me about a barnyard surgery case that Dr. Harris performed.

"It was a cold winter night. The cow had to have a caesarean if she was going to make it. We drove her into the back stall and stretched her out on her side between two support posts. Dr. Harris had a young kid acting as his surgical assistant along with him. I guess that's what you call it. Anyway, the cow was in bad shape, but Dr. Harris was doing what he could. It wasn't his fault. The boy's name was Rick, I think. Dr. Harris would ask Rick to provide him with the appropriate piece of equipment, just like on the television. The poor cow wasn't doing any good. Finally she started breathing her last. It would have been tragic if it hadn't been so funny. Dr. Harris was on top of the situation. 'Rick,' he called, 'sledge hammer, please.' Rick looked nonplused, Dr. Harris mockingly serious, but I had to burst out laughing in spite of the circumstances. Yes, sir, Dr. Harris always had a sense of humor. Sure sorry he's sick and hope he gets well. We need him around here."

"I'm sure he will." After putting the equipment back in the car trunk, I said good-night and returned to town.

The next morning, Wednesday, John was again awaiting me at the table, cigar in one hand and coffee cup in the other. "Jim, I'm ready to get on the road. Got the adrenalin flowing."

"Dr. Wilkerson told you to stay off the road," reminded Sally.

"I heard him but that don't keep me from being ready to go. Jim, Howard and I are going to work together and feed you calls as you go. This ought to be an eighteen-call day for you. Just don't waste time visiting with the farmers; they don't pay for conversation time. And, Jim, please, don't sightsee as you go. Floorboard that accelerator. You're losing too much time between stops."

Sally was standing in the door behind John. I could see her shaking her head negatively as John was talking about floorboarding the accelerator. I smiled and assured John I would do my best. After eating, I got on the way.

Howard and John did work together that day. I think they had some of those calls that are "stop when you're in the neighborhood" up their sleeves. I had no dairy herd tests to delay me. By the time I returned to the house that evening, I had indeed made sixteen stops and, with still the evening to go, it appeared that John's magic number might be within reach.

"Jim, you're learning. I'm going to make a million-dollar man out of you yet," John greeted me on my arrival.

"I wouldn't count on that."

"You made sixteen calls, didn't you?"

"Yes, but . . ."

"Now, Jim, it was speed between stops. I was calling the wives at each stop and timing you."

"That was dedication on your part."

"Better than watching soap operas, Jim. Jim, I figured that you averaged fifty miles per hour between stops today. That's a lot better than you must have been doing."

"I guess I was driving a little faster."

"Jim, it's speed that counts. Time between calls is wasted time. Remember that, and you'll make that million dollars."

"John, the problem is that the western part of my practice is range country. There are far fewer ranch houses in such areas; thus the distance between stops is far greater. Here, you have an average of two houses per section; there, I have one house per two or three sections. Anyway, why don't you increase the margin on your medicine. You could slow down then. Probably your speeding tickets are eating into your profits anyway. Profits from medicine sales don't depend on speed. Why don't you try it?"

"You didn't hear about Bill Smith, the veterinarian over in the neighboring county, trying to compete in medicine prices with me?"

"I guess not. My practice is 150 miles away."

"No, I guess you wouldn't have heard. Well, Bill thought I was making too much money so he tried to move in on me. He rented an empty filling station building on the highway east of town. Stocked it with medicines and put a person in there to take calls for him and to peddle medicines."

"He did? How did he come out?"

"I'm still here, aren't I? I just told Howard to drop my medicine costs down to my purchase costs. Had Bill closing up that station within ninety days. No, Jim, I could raise prices of medicines, but I've got competitors just waiting for a chance to pounce."

I couldn't argue with logic so changed the subject. After supper I excused myself so I could complete the day's work and make the magic eighteen calls.

The next morning John was elated. After breakfast he escorted me to the door and put me on the road with words of encouragement to go out and see if I couldn't beat the eighteen-call record I had established for myself the previous day. I returned to the house that evening with only thirteen calls behind me.

"Been a bad day, Jim. Just couldn't get things organized."

"John, I have a two-way radio in my car. It sure helps on communicating with my office."

"Can't afford it, Jim. Telephone charges are cheaper. You're out in the big pasture country and miles between stops. It might pay for you but not here."

"Maybe so."

As I was eating, John continued talking. "Jim, I've been doing some pencil and paper work today while you were in the country."

"That better than watching the soap operas?"

"You bet. One day of that was enough. Jim, I've got news for you. You can't make a million dollars in your practice area. Too much distance between stops. Cattle just aren't worth that much."

"I'd figured that out about ten years ago, John."

"Jim, you and Marian ought to move up to one of the adjoining counties and practice. Farms are smaller, so you don't waste time driving."

"You'd probably run me out of business even in a neighboring county."

"You're probably right, Jim. I just don't show mercy to competitors."

The next morning John went into the office as I left for the country. "Dr. Wilkerson didn't say I couldn't go to the office. I had Howard line up some dogs for me to spay and some others to vaccinate that were on the wait list."

That night John was in good spirits. I had handled fifteen calls and he had spayed four dogs and vaccinated about ten more.

"I can still find those ovaries, Jim. If I wanted to I could give those other dog and cat vets in town a run for their money."

"I'm sure you could. It would be wise for you to slow down and share the wealth. You've just about earned your second million, you said."

"Jim, I'm going to earn that third million."

In the following conversation we agreed that I would return to my home the next morning, Saturday. John was feeling well again and he had Dr. Wilkerson's permission to go back to work.

On my trip home I kept remembering John's words that my ranch practice had too much traveling involved—that I just wasn't going to make a million dollars. Maybe, I thought, it would just be nice to retire to a salaried job with a pension—especially one in an area with warm breezes and palm trees.

"Marian, How Would You Like to Live on a Tropical Island?"

A veterinarian, like the family doctor at that time, was supposed to be on call at any hour. When one was sick, this was easier said than done.

"Junior, is that you?" I was sick. It was 8:30 P.M. and I just wasn't enthusiastic about going out again. Maybe I could stall this caller until tomorrow or . . .

"This is Sally Perkins. I live down in Coon Hollow, remember?"

"Sure, I remember." Sally was a widow lady who stayed on the farm after her husband's death. Her sons rented the land and did the farm work, but Sally still kept a few head of livestock and some chickens to keep herself in meat, eggs, and pin money, as she said. Coon Hollow, where she lived, was in a canyon that led down from the uplands into the river bottom land below. I remembered Coon Hollow all too well. On a trip out there two years before, my car had skidded off the muddy road that led down into the canyon. I had to walk three-quarters of a mile to a neighbor's to get him to come over with his tractor and pull me back on the road. It had been raining all day. The road into Sally's place would again be muddy.

"My steer hasn't been eating very good today. He's going into my locker come fall to feed me through the winter. I just can't afford to have anything happen to him. Junior, can you come out?"

"Well, Mrs. Perkins, I'm not feeling good myself. Couldn't it wait until morning?"

"I just wouldn't be able to sleep tonight worrying about it. I think you'd better come out now."

"But, Mrs. Perkins, your road will be in bad shape. I don't think I ought to try it after dark. Remember the last time I was out at your place?"

"Now, Junior, if you keep on the inside of the road next to the bluff you won't slip off. The road is passable. As least it drains well so you won't get mired down. Just keep on the inside and you'll make it all right."

"But, Mrs. Perkins, I am running a fever. I really should stay home this evening."

"Now, Junior, you come on out. The steer needs attention tonight."

I wasn't going to get out of it. "O.K., Mrs. Perkins, I'll be out. Look for me in about thirty minutes."

As I drove out I began to analyze my circumstances. Here I was a college graduate working sometimes round the clock even when I was sick. Many times, and probably this time, I was sicker than the creature I was being called to doctor. I was getting close to forty years of age. If I was going to change my work, I should change before I was forty. I had to make up my mind.

Still pondering the question—the question that was to occupy my mind intermittently for the next couple of years—I crept successfully down the road that ran into Coon Hollow and Sally Perkins's place. Sally came out to meet me carrying a lantern.

"The steer is here in the barn. I kept him up so you could see him tonight." She led me into the barn and to a box stall in which she had confined the animal.

I followed along behind. I was feverish but that was usual this time of year. It was just that I didn't seem to have the stamina to keep going when it got dark. She hung the lantern up and opened the stall gate to admit me. I stood there by the gate observing the steer.

"Mrs. Perkins, this steer is chewing its cud. What makes you think it's sick?"

"Junior, he just isn't eating today like he should. He didn't clean up the feed I gave him. I feed him separately from the others since I'm fattening him. That way I know how much he eats."

"But, Mrs. Perkins, he sure doesn't look sick. Maybe you just put more feed out today."

"No, the same amount. I measure it out in a gallon can so I know exactly what he gets. No, he's sick. I know it."

I wasn't going to get out of it that easy, it seemed. I slipped the lariat I was carrying over the steer's head and fastened him in the corner. Next I took a thermometer from the case I carried in my shirt pocket and examined it under the lantern light to see what it read. It read 102°F, so I shook it down with a few vigorous swings of my arm and examined it again. It read just above 98°F then, so I stepped around behind the steer and inserted the thermometer into the anus of the steer, taking care that a portion was protruding so that I could later extract it to read the temperature. When I did so the temperature read 101.4°F.

"The steer's temperature is normal." I told Sally what the temperature read.

"Well, he's sick. I know that. Maybe he ate some jimsonweed. There's some out in the lot and it's the only thing that's come up this spring yet. They won't run a fever with jimsonweed poisoning, will they?"

"I don't think he would be chewing his cud if he was poisoned."

"Now I don't know. Armer treated a steer I had back in '47 or maybe it was '46. Anyway it was the same year that Alfred—Alfred was my husband, you know—it was the same year he died. That steer chewed its cud up until the time it dropped over dead."

I wasn't going to get out of it by that approach. I was still Junior to the older generation—and was still living under Armer's shadow. I listened to the steer's heart and lungs and kneaded his rumen. Everything was apparently normal. God, here I was sick and should be in bed. I needed to rest to be able to go tomorrow. Instead I was out looking at a healthy animal just to placate an elderly lady. Somehow it seemed like my rest was more important than hers tonight.

"Well, Mrs. Perkins, let's give him a laxative and I'll leave you a tonic you can pour on his feed every day. I'm sure he'll be all right." I proceeded to mix up some medicine in a bucket of water and pumped it down into the steer's stomach with some assistance from Sally. Next I dispensed a small bottle of medicine to her and explained the dosage as I wrote the directions on the label.

"You don't think you ought to be giving him some of that penicillin stuff, Junior? I don't want him to die. I don't know what I would eat next winter if he did."

"No, I don't think he needs any antibiotics. Just watch him. If he isn't all right in a day or two, let me know." After collecting my bill, I got back into my car and started back towards town.

On the way back to town, in my mind I began to call the roll of my classmates. Fully a third of them were holding down salaried jobs with the government, with institutions, or with industry. They were probably doing as well as myself, if not better, considering the fringe benefits, and weren't having to work at night. Another third of my classmates were engaged in small animal practice. There, too, they were able to lead reasonably regulated lives and certainly profited far more than myself. I had enjoyed the work during my early years in practice. It was no longer enjoyable—at least at night when I didn't feel well. At the same time the clients were entitled to veterinary service around the clock when needed. It wasn't fair to them not to have an able-bodied veterinarian in the area. My mind began to contemplate other types of work.

"Marian, how would you like to move to a South Sea island?" I asked when I crawled into bed.

"You've got a fever," she replied.

"How about Tahiti? It doesn't get cold there."

"Sure, why not?"

At least the seed was planted. I pulled the covers up around my neck and envisioned hula dancers on tropical beaches as I drifted off into a feverish sleep.

DATE DUE

SEP 27 '86	FEB 13 '87		
OCT 6 '86	APR 13 1987		
OCT 8 '86	AUG 22 '88		
OCT 8 '86	SEP 5 '89		
OCT 8 '86	JUL 2 '90		
OCT 27 '86			
NOV 18 '86			
NOV 30 '86			
DEC 26 '86			
JAN 13 '87			
JAN 27 '87			
FEB 2 '87			